Table of Co

CW00457659

Section 1 ....

Why Bodyweight Training? ....

Health Check ....

Where To Start With Bodyweight Training? 8

Types Of Bodyweight Training 14

Master The Basics Before Anything Else 18

The "Big 5" Progression Path 21

Abs And Core 23

Negative & Eccentric Training 31

Isometrics 33

Exercise Equipment? 39

The Warm Up 43

Your Personalised Training Plan 45

Exercise Routines 57

Section 2 70

Introduction to section 2 71

The Exercises 72

Push Ups Progression 73

Pullups Progression 82

Dips Progression 89

Shoulder Press Progression 96

Bodyweight Squats Progression 107

Abdominal & lower back exercises 118

Upper abs 119

Lower abs 132

Lower back 145

Thank you! If you found this useful, I'd like to help further... 158

Remember The Podcast! 160

Cardio Training. 161

Also by James Atkinson 165

Blank Program Cards 168

JimsHealthAndMuscle.com

Bodyweight Training

&

Calisthenics

The Progressive Bodyweight Workout Book

For Beginners & Beyond

James Atkinson

Section 1

Why Bodyweight Training?

Bodyweight training:

- Can be used by anyone.
- Increases strength.
- Develops mobility.
- Increases muscular control.
- Burns fat.
- Provides an amazing (if not the best) foundation for resistance training.
- Helps you identify weaknesses.
- Is the most practical form of resistance training.
- Can lead to some very impressive party tricks. ☺

What will you learn?

How to progress from zero to advanced trainer with "the big 5":

- Push-ups.
- Pullups.
- Dips.
- Shoulder press.
- Squats.

Other essential elements and progression, such as

- Core strength and abdominal development.
- Negatives and eccentric bodyweight training.
- Isometrics explained.
- How to create and plan your own bodyweight training routine.

You will learn how to create your very own bodyweight training routine based on your current ability. There are resources included and a walkthrough guide that you can follow to ensure that you have the most efficient training plan that will set you up for progression right away.

BODYWEIGHT TRAINING & CALISTHENICS

Let's imagine you are a beginner to resistance training and you want to develop muscle strength, tone, and functionality. What's the most practical first step? Join a gym? Buy some home workout equipment? Hire a personal trainer?

Let's also flip the coin and imagine that you are no stranger to resistance training and have a good level of fitness, but have, for whatever reason, decided that you would like to look into bodyweight training. What should you do as a starting point? Do you go right ahead and acquire a set of paralletts, dip, pull up bars or some kind of suspension kit?

My answer to this question whether you are a beginner or not is to utilise what you already have. Of course you can travel the path of the above ideas and can absolutely have great success in any training method but bodyweight training is by far the most practical for beginners and veterans alike as all you need is your body, gravity and a bit of knowledge to challenge yourself and get on the fitness progression ladder.

The aim of this book is to give you the knowledge and toolkit to not only be able to competently train with bodyweight and calisthenics exercises, but to also spark your creativity to try new things and progress effectively towards your fitness goals.

Bodyweight training is an excellent choice of resistance training for almost everyone. For the beginner or senior trainer it can be an entry point to fitness that will yield unbelievable results as bodyweight exercise is often more than enough to challenge previously unconditioned muscle groups with progressive overload, leading to results that can be superior to the same intensity of training from barbells and dumbbells, etc. In my experience, I believe that this is because of the functional nature of bodyweight training and calisthenics that lend itself to core stability, along with a bigger emphasis on our stabiliser muscles.

For the veteran of exercise, bodyweight training is an excellent supplement to an existing fitness routine as it can add another dimension to fitness progression, refresh a stagnant programme, and even send the trainer on a new exciting path. Another value of bodyweight training for the veteran is that it can highlight weaknesses.

For the best part of thirty years, I've been involved in resistance training one way or the other. Strength training, bodybuilding and endurance have been part of my life at some point. Throughout this time, I have increasingly prioritised exercise form and everything that goes with this, such as control and range of movement over anything else.

So if exercise form is the number one priority when it comes to resistance training, I can tell you that bodyweight training is an excellent foundation for everyone. This way of training and the mind-set that goes along with it will greatly enhance everything else you decide to do.

For example, if you build up from not being able to perform a singly chin up to being able to complete a set of eight or more in good form, and then decide that you want to become a bodybuilder, you will have an enormous advantage and be way ahead of the trainer that has the same goal as you but visits the gym as their first step.

Why? Because you will have built strength, control and muscle in your latissimus dorsi (back muscles), your mobility will be good, your core and stabiliser muscles will be more developed and more equipped to protect and assist you with heavier weights and you will have the stamina to use progressive overload to good effect.

If you look at all the experts in bodyweight training, you notice they are very well defined, with lean, solid bodies. This is no accident, as bodyweight training and calisthenics really do promote fat burning. During your exercise sessions, you will hold static poses that engage multiple muscle groups, often pushing these to exhaustion, or you will perform very controlled reps that also push multiple muscle groups to exhaustion. It's no secret that the more energy that you exert, the more lean muscle you develop, the more calories you will burn and this is the bottom line here.

The more you train with this method, the more your body will adapt, so if you fully commit to it, you progress and challenge yourself. You can expect to develop a similar, lean and solid physique to these bodyweight training experts.

One of the biggest draws for some people to bodyweight training and calisthenics is the amount of amazing and impressive tricks you can develop! Who doesn't want to know someone that can do a set of handstand push-ups, muscle ups, human flag, muscle ups or the Planche? Although these movements are impressive to look at, they are still exercises that need much development in form and muscle function. So if you are getting into this, I would suggest that you have a goal of achieving something special like this and work towards it by understanding what it takes to achieve and taking the steps to get there. Although we will not cover these specialist movements in this book, everything that is covered forms the foundation for these feats of strengths.

My name is James Atkinson (Jim to my readers and friends). I've been into fitness and exercise for most of my life and my experience has an extreme range, from skinny to competing bodybuilder, from fat to endurance runner, I have formal qualifications in advanced fitness instruction, and I'm an Amazon bestselling author in the fitness niche.

This information is not an excuse for me to brag, but I believe it's essential for you to know some background on the author of potential exercise advice that you intend to follow. At this point, I want to thank you for your purchase and let you know I am always willing to help where I can with your fitness journey.

I'd also like you to know that I am a real person, (not a ghost writer) I'm passionate about my subject and write from personal experience, I have had great success with fitness but part of the journey to great success was often great failure and I have that too. If I can share relevant, personal experiences of my failures to help you avoid potential problems, then this is no failure!

The bottom line is that I want you to get results and I'm here to help you get to where you want to be in fitness! If you are not where you want to be and can't see a path, I have a free podcast where I chat about common issues and give advice on how to overcome and progress. Get a coffee on, drop by and have a listen at:

AudioFitTest.com

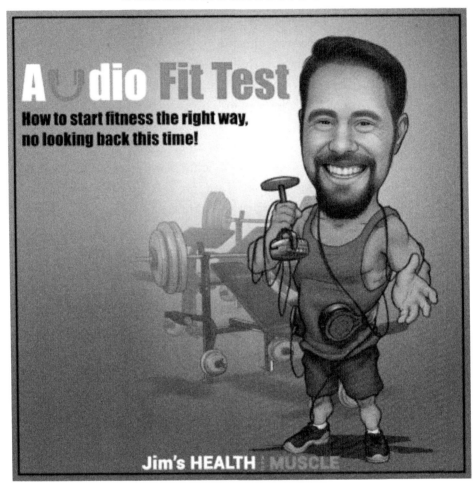

Health Check

Before you embark on any fitness routine, please consult your Doctor or physiotherapist. If you have any health conditions, always check if the type of exercise and exercise choices you intend to involve yourself with.

1. Do not exercise if you are unwell.

2. Stop if you feel pain, and if the pain does not subside, consult your Doctor or physiotherapist.

3. Do not exercise if you have taken alcohol or had a large meal in the last few hours.

4. If you are taking medication, please check with your Doctor to make sure it is okay for you to exercise.

5. If in doubt at all, please check with your Doctor or physiotherapist first – you may even want to take this routine and go through it with them. It may be helpful to ask for a blood pressure, cholesterol and weight check. You can then have these taken again in a few months to see the benefit.

Where To Start With Bodyweight Training?

Bodyweight exercise can be very difficult, and it's easy to get inspired by others that are doing some amazing things with pull up bars, rings or even with no equipment, but these amazing feats of strength are not things that just happen. In most cases, they result from a progressive approach.

The good news is that working towards a bodyweight training effect or a specific goal with bodyweight exercise is easy to start.

The first thing that should be understood with bodyweight training is that it is essentially just another form of resistance training. All this means is that you are resisting a force against gravity.

At the time of writing, gravity is constant, so it always stays the same. The variable that you do have the ability to easily change is the force that you work with.

It's easy to understand this basic rule, but with body mechanics, there is more to learn. Already in this guide I've talked about the importance of exercise form and this is something I make a big noise about in all of my other fitness books, but it has a direct link to the "gravity and force thing" and to the "body mechanics thing".

Learn your basic kinesiology:

Kinesiology is the movement and function of the human body. A simple example of this is if you were to hold your arms out to your sides so they are straight and parallel to the floor, you understand that your shoulder joint is raised and that your lateral deltoid (mid shoulder muscle) is the main muscle being worked or "challenged against gravity":

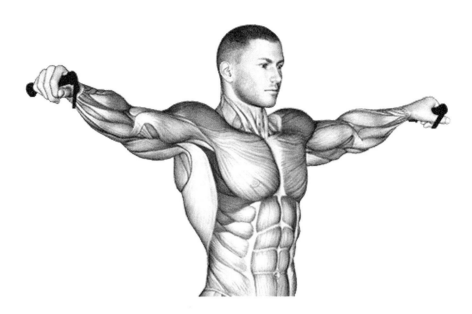

Another example is if you stand up straight, bend over at the waist so your upper body is at a slight angle to the floor, bring your elbows up so that your upper arms are parallel with the floor and then straighten your lower arms, you will know firstly that your abs and lower back are engaged by keeping you in this position, but with the arm movement, you will target your triceps:

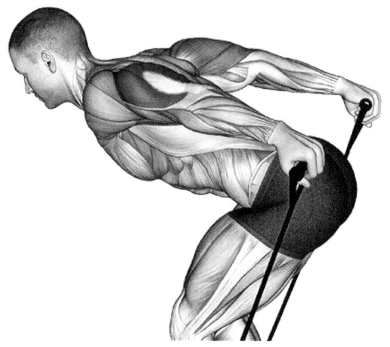

These are examples of movements that your body is designed to perform. They may not look like movements that are used in everyday life, but I feel it's a really valuable exercise for everyone to become aware of which muscles are used in movement and joint function.

Having a basic understanding of kinesiology in this way will greatly improve the effectiveness of your training sessions, help you get the most out of your workouts and help you strive for perfect exercise form.

This stuff will not only benefit you in bodyweight training and calisthenics, but it's invaluable for every type of resistance training that you may get involved in, and will also impact the way you approach physical activities in everyday life.

At the base level, there are seven major body parts that we all use for everyday life and for fitness. How much do you know about how to target these with resistance and movement?

I know you didn't sign up for this, but here's a thinking exercise if you feel like testing yourself! ☺

Name an exercise choice or movement that targets your:

- Chest
- Back
- Legs
- Biceps
- Shoulders
- Triceps
- Abs

Learning exercise choices and knowing simple kinesiology in order to target muscle groups you want to develop actually comes with practical experience, research and, at the highest level, formal qualifications. You can, however, gain a basic understanding of which muscle groups are worked when you move your body in different ways during everyday life. And it certainly builds good awareness if you think about this when you are performing normal activities.

A fine example of this that I have seen repeatedly with clients wanting to get into fitness or clients that have weak glutes and leg muscles and would like to develop these muscle groups is that they neglect to use them in everyday life.

If I am asked for advice on how to build, shape or tone weak glutes or legs, the first thing I will do here is to take a regular chair and ask that they sit down as they normally would. Sound strange? Well, sitting on a chair from a standing position means that you have to perform the start of a squat, this means that if you were conscious of the muscle groups used in everyday life, you could easily engage your glutes and quads every time you took a seat and the same in reverse when leaving the seat.

If you look at the way someone who has underdeveloped glutes and quads sits down on a chair, in most cases you will see that the chair is used to break their fall as a priority and is something to sit on as its secondary role. So if the client is now told about the function of the glutes and legs and the benefits of squats as an exercise choice, we can start to develop the squat technique. The first step in learning to squat is engaging the muscles that are used to sit on a chair so. This can be done outside the gym in everyday life, so awareness of these muscles and this action can be taken away by the client.

Sticking with leg function, another problem that can lead to weaker quads and leg muscles that many people have is when in a standing position; it's common to lock the knees to take away the effort of using the quads for stabilisation. This means that the quads will not be engaged as they should. So if the awareness of this is highlighted to someone, when they are in a standing position, cooking, waiting in a queue, washing up, etc. A slight bend in the knees to engage the quads will help to develop these muscles very quickly.

These are some examples of fairly basic rules, but practicing them and learning to be aware of them will greatly improve workout technique, effectiveness and vastly improve the speed of development in these muscle groups.

If you are in this group and decide to take this on board and give it a go, you might find it pretty uncomfortable at first but the more you do it, the better you will be and the easier it will be until it becomes second nature.

Learning kinesiology and muscle function is an ongoing process, and it's something that you should always look to be improving on. This goes for bodyweight training and every other form of fitness, and the best way to become familiar with this is to start working out with the awareness.

Having a strong base to work with is the next step, and following a basic resistance program that uses compound movements will certainly give you this. You can simply go to a gym, grab some resistance bands and train with what I like to call the "bread and butter compound movements".

Compound exercises are king for building stability and strength effectively and here is the list of movements that I would recommend training with for each muscle group. Yes, this is the answer to the question above ☺

- Chest: A chest press such as push ups, bench press with resistance bands, barbells, dumbbells or a chest press machine
- Back: A row such as reverse push ups, pull ups, lat pull down, rows with resistance bands, barbells, dumbbells or a row machine
- Legs: A leg press such as squats using bodyweight, resistance bands, barbells, dumbbells or a leg press machine
- Biceps: Bicep curls with barbells, dumbbells, resistance bands
- Shoulders: A shoulder press such as a variation of handstand push ups or using resistance bands, barbells or dumbbells
- Triceps: A tricep extension or dip such any variation of dip, tricep pushdowns, overhead tricep extensions with resistance bands,

dumbbells or barbells
- Abs: A crunch such as a variation of crunches on the floor or with a machine

Triceps, biceps and abs are muscle groups that don't really have many options for compound exercise choices because of the mechanics of the body, but I think it's sensible to single these muscle groups out to ensure they are getting challenged.

When working exclusively with compound exercises, it's not uncommon to ignore these muscle groups or work them in as less of a priority. The reason for this is that biceps, triceps, and abs are actually used as "synergists" in many other exercises. For example, with any chest press, push up, etc. The triceps are also challenged and, with any row movement, the biceps are bought into the exercise. Depending on the intensity of these lifts and the goal or the trainer, there may not be any need to single these muscle groups out.

With exercise routines that do include triceps, biceps and abs, it's a sensible choice to add these in towards the end of the workout as this way, all other exercises that use these muscles as synergists will be performed without the possibility of fatigue.

Depending on your ability or progression with basic strength training, if you want to achieve something special with bodyweight training such as hand stand push ups or the planch, you can start training towards this goal by actually doing. After all, there is no better way to achieve something than actually doing that thing.

Even if you have developed a good foundation in strength training, you will still need to take small steps to achieve a big goal like this, but you will have a big advantage that will get you over the finish line a lot quicker and easier. This is covered later in the guide.

Types Of Bodyweight Training

Using your bodyweight to target a specific muscle group can be defined in many ways, and there is certainly more than one way to train with your own bodyweight.

Exercise methods such as pilates and yoga are excellent forms of bodyweight training, offer many benefits and should never be overlooked.

I have always seen exercise methods such as yoga and pilates as a "supplement" to a resistance program. This type of exercise will almost always benefit every type of trainer, offering them a better understanding of kinesiology as explained earlier and the ability to understand body function. Pilates and yoga also help individuals to identify personal weakness or problem areas that have the potential to affect any other resistance training that they do.

An example of my personal experience and appreciation for this type of exercise started when I was invited to be a case study for a pilates student during their formal training. I agreed to be treated as a total beginner to fitness and the study began.

During the several weeks of assessment and progressive training, we quickly highlighted a weakness that I had that was affecting my usual resistance training. I mentioned that sometimes I would suffer from lower back pain. During my early weight lifting days many years ago, I had slipped a disk in my lower back and this would always come back to haunt me every now and again if I pushed myself too hard or had a momentary slip in concentration with my exercise form. The injury is something that I've learned to manage well and it never really holds me back, so I didn't see it as a problem.

When working with resistance exercises, I've always strived to maintain excellent exercise form and one of the fundamental rules is to "keep your abs tight" during your lifts, so this was second nature to me. During my pilates experience, I was introduced to something called "diaphragmatic breathing" and this changed the way I "kept my abs tight" from then on.

It turned out that I was doing a good job of keeping my abs tight throughout my resistance training, but I was neglecting the lower abs. This meant that my lower, deep abs were weaker than the rest of them, which meant that my lower back was not being supported as well as it could have been. From that point on, I have worked on this new "keeping my abs tight" method and had zero back pain issues!

From my brief introduction into pilates, I not only learned something new about my strengths and weaknesses but also learned how to prevent the occasional back pain. It was very reassuring to learn that the back injury I sustained all those years ago was not actually the problem.

So if you get the opportunity to work with a pilates or yoga teacher that's experienced and passionate about their subject, you should definitely take it up.

There are two ways of exercising with bodyweight covered in this book, and these are calisthenics and isometric training. The difference between these when compared to pilates and yoga is that calisthenics and isometric training have a strong focus on muscular strength and growth. The reason for covering both calisthenics and isometric training is that the training methods overlap nicely and can be used in conjunction with each other.

Calisthenics

Calisthenics is a form of training using bodyweight exercises to stimulate muscle groups through a certain range of movement. For this book, we will consider calisthenics to be:

"Bodyweight exercise that has a dynamic form, using more than one joint movement,"

Calisthenics in is an old word that originated in Greece, and the practical idea of it was to use bodyweight movements to create strength in the muscles along with an aesthetically pleasing physique. This is a great goal to have for anyone who shows an interest in their health and wellbeing.

Calisthenics training usually uses the number of repetitions of an exercise ("reps") to measure progression and ability.

Isometrics

Isometric training is a form of resistance training in which the body is held statically in varying positions to stimulate muscle groups. For this guide, we will consider isometric training to be:

"Bodyweight exercise that has a static form to strengthen varying muscle groups,"

There are two ways to work with isometric training. The first is to use your bodyweight against gravity, and the other is to push or pull against something. This could be against your own body using your strength or you could use a solid, stationary platform like a wall.

Isometric training usually uses "time spent" in a position as the measure of progression and ability.

6 to 10 second holds when pushing/ pulling at maximum effort is a sensible start with isometrics and this timescale can be seen as the equivalent to "1 rep" of a calisthenics exercise. This is useful to know when it comes to planning your workouts.

Many instructors will class all types of bodyweight exercise as calisthenics, but I believe it's valuable to be able to differentiate between callisthenic and isometric training, as there are differences. But with that said, both calisthenics and isometric training fit together excellently.

Master The Basics Before Anything Else

I was around fifteen years old when I first got invited to visit a weight lifting gym. I'd been playing rugby for several years and had been getting better at the game at this time. But it was becoming very apparent that I was not developing as fast as my teammates and, indeed, the guys on the teams that we played against. Everyone was getting bigger and stronger than me, which left me at a disadvantage. I'd get thrown around on the pitch and even in training to the point where it must have felt pretty dangerous for the coaches to give me a position on the team. This meant that I had to sit on the bench as a substitute in every game and this was extremely disheartening for me, as rugby was a genuine passion of mine.

Luckily for me, one of my neighbours and friend of the family was a power lifter. He suggested I get into powerlifting to build strength and size, and that I could start going with him to the gym so he could teach me how to lift.

This would be great! In a few weeks I'd be a hulk on the rugby pitch that no one could take down and I'd be hard to replace in the team! After all, I didn't know anyone else that lifted weights, or anyone else who had someone to teach them!

So we headed to the gym on a Sunday evening. As soon as I stepped through the door, the first thing I noticed were the chunky barbells, racks and heavy plates all lined up. There were some big guys doing squats with heavy barbells that were bending with the weight of the plates and it was very clear that this was definitely the environment you should be in if you wanted to develop real strength and size.

After my new mentor had said hello to a few of these guys and introduced me as "the next Jonah Lomu" (Maybe my introduction to sarcasm), he took me to one of the squat racks that wasn't in use. This thing had an Olympic bar (weighing 20kg as standard), a bench and plenty of heavy iron discs to load up the bar with.

"Squats are going to be your bread and butter here, a brilliant exercise for strong, powerful legs, so let's start with squats."

My coach said as he moved the bench out of the way so we could get right into it.

He stepped underneath the bar so it rested across the back of his shoulders and traps and casually stood up straight to un-rack it and stepped back. He then took me through the movement, explaining the benefits of the squat and how to perform the exercise before re-racking it and giving me my first opportunity to try.

I did as he had and performed a set of squats to the best of my ability under my mentor's guidance. Once the bar was re-racked, I could see he was thinking.

"You really need to strengthen your glutes and your hamstrings are a bit tight, so let's work on the form for the next few weeks. Go and grab one of those and let's have another go."

He said as he pointed to a corner of the gym. Against the wall right next to a poster of Arnold flexing his biceps with the caption "Keep on pumping" was a stack of wooden bars the same length as the Olympic bar I had just lifted.

I headed over there and picked one up. This was basically a long version of a broom handle.

So I was in a power lifting gym learning to squat, deadlift, bench press and shoulder press with a broom handle and it didn't half knock my confidence, to where I didn't look forward to going to the gym in the early days. But I knew if I wanted to play rugby again, I would have to.

Several months later, I could squat 60kg for 10 reps with good form and it progressed very quickly from there.

What's my point? Before I knew anything about lifting weights; I thought that the first time I visited the gym, I would actually be lifting weights, not a wooden bar. In reality, I had to learn the basics, and learn them well, before I could progress to the good stuff.

Knowing what I know now, this was the very best introduction to the world of resistance training that I could have had, and this is one of the most fundamental rules about any form of fitness that I always make extra effort to highlight.

Bodyweight training is no exception. If you want to excel at this, you should learn to master the basic movements before moving onto the advanced stuff.

The basic movements in bodyweight training are very similar to that of powerlifting in that they are compound movements and they use the same mechanics.

Your first goal in bodyweight training is to learn these exercises and be able to perform the rep range that goes with each one in good form before moving on. I call these exercises "the big 5".

- Standard Push-up – 20 reps
- Standard Pullups – 10 reps
- Dips – 15 reps
- Shoulder press – 15 reps
- Bodyweight squats – 20 reps

Everyone who starts calisthenics starts from a different point regarding ability and fitness level, so for some, this will be easier to achieve than for others. If you are very new to fitness and are starting from scratch, this may look daunting or impossible to achieve, but I can assure you that with the correct build up, you can progress faster than you think.

If you can't do a single push up, pullups look like an impossibility and you haven't got a clue how to even do a shoulder press with just body weight, this is no problem!

We have covered the steps in this guide that you can take in order to sensibly work towards, achieve, and progress far beyond this goal.

Some of these progressions require that you invest in some small, inexpensive pieces of training equipment. It's always good to have some form of exercise band handy if you are into fitness, as these will come in handy for all types of fitness training. So grab yourself an exercise band set or an equivalent. You will need a few lengths to get started. There are also many variations of dip bars and pull up bars widely available that are designed for use in the home, so grab some of these as well.

The "Big 5" Progression Path

Before getting right into full on calisthenics, isometric training and negative reps (all covered later in the guide), it's really important that we learn to walk before we can run, and this goes for every type of new skill and fitness method.

If you are new to exercise and find it hard to complete over 20 reps of standard push-ups, 10 standard pull ups etc, you will need to take some steps to work towards this. With exercise and fitness, there are always challenges and progressions, so knowing where you are in relation to your goal is the first step, but knowing how to take the correct actions to work towards your goals is the next step. This is what we will cover in this section.

It's a well-known fact that if you want to get better at something, you need to do more of that thing. But if you can't do that thing, it's pretty tricky to put this into action. If you struggle with one, or any of the "big 5" exercises mentioned in the previous chapter, this chapter will guide you through the process of progression to being able to achieve this goal and move on to more exciting and impressive bodyweight training later.

This should be where everyone wishing to start calisthenics and bodyweight training begins, as it will develop a strong foundation for future progress, making it easier and quicker to transition to more challenging goals.

There are several progressions to each of these "big 5" exercises that you can follow. Each exercise has an illustration of the start and mid positions, a written description and a suggestion on how to use the exercise in order to work towards the next progression.

The list of progressions is as follows:
Standard Push Ups

- Standing push ups
- Incline push ups
- Standard push ups
- Push ups with bars

Standard Pullups

- Incline rows
- Engage and hang
- Standard pullups

Standard Dips

- Assisted dips
- Seated dips
- Standard dips

Standard Shoulder Press

- Standing incline press
- Incline press
- Pike press
- Elevated pike press
- Standard shoulder press

Bodyweight Squats

- Seat squats
- Bodyweight squats
- Elevated pistol squats
- Pistol squats

You will find these exercises in "The Exercises" section of the book.

Abs And Core

Having a strong core is essential not only for bodyweight training, but will also be beneficial for every other form of fitness, exercise and everyday life activities. Because of the nature of calisthenics, this resistance training method gives us strength in the abdominals and hip flexors by default, provided that our exercise form of these basic movements is good.

Most (if not all) bodyweight exercises require an engagement of the abs and core to perform, so they are used as "synergists" and "stabilisers" for pretty much every exercise.

With this said, the key word here is "engagement". There is a difference between engaging a muscle and working it through its full range of motion, and abdominals are no different to any other muscle group.

If you decide to leave out any kind of exercise that specifically targets the abdominals and their full range of motion, in favour of focusing on everything else, your abs will become strong enough to support your form with every other exercise you do, and if you stay lean by keeping your body fat percentage to a minimum, they will be visible. But this will neglect to bring in the abdominal muscles full potential.

Rather than settling for a set of abs that are strong as synergists and stabilisers only, why not work them to their full potential and build a truly solid core? If you can build a set of abdominals that are strong in every way that they were designed to function, you will progress much faster, have better control, and be functionally solid through your entire core.

Where do you start with extra focus on the abs and core to single them out for greater strength and function? As it is with the "Big 5" exercises, there are also progressions to work on in this area.

In this section, we will look at a selection of abdominal and core exercises and highlight how to approach effective abdominal workouts, along with a bit of mechanical advice on how the abs and core are targeted.

I have always found it useful to look at the abs in two parts, the upper section and the lower section, and for a solid all over abs workout, you should target both areas. One rule that is super helpful in figuring out which abs exercises target which area is:

If your legs are being drawn up towards your chests, this is a lower abs exercise. If your head and chest are being drawn towards your legs, it's an upper abs exercise.

Of course, either type of ab exercise will have an engagement of both the upper and lower, but if you want to target either part of the abs individually, you can follow this rule.

An example of an upper ab exercise is the well-known "Crunch" or "Sit up" and an example of a lower ab exercise is the "knee raise".

Another very important rule that I believe doesn't get anywhere near enough emphasis when it comes to abs workouts is that to work abs properly, you need the range of movement. We have touched on range of movement already, but what does this mean and how do you put the abs through their full range of movement?

If abdominal muscles are the same as any other muscle, this means they have a full extension and a maximum contraction position. If you know and understand how to do this, you can avoid the mistake that many people make when working out their abs.

Let's look at the maximum contraction position for the lower abs by using the example, hanging knee raises.

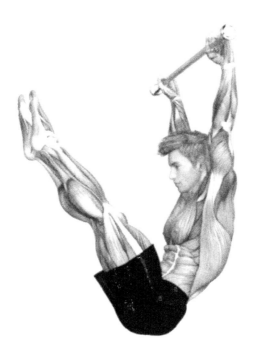

The picture above shows the maximum contraction position for hanging knee raises. This is the point where the abdominals are at their "top of movement". The big take away is that at this position, the lower spine is flexed because the hips are tilted. One of the most common mistakes in abdominal exercises is not tilting the hips to flex the spine.

If the spine is not flexed, deep muscles called hip flexors will be the main muscles being worked, taking away the range of movement and workload from the abdominals themselves.

So an upper abs exercise is the basic crunch. This is how you get the maximum range of movement in this area.

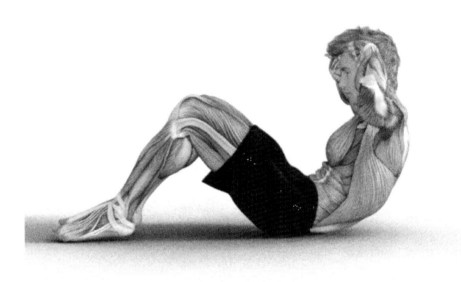

The main point here is that you keep your lower back flat and pushed into the floor or bench. This way, you will transfer all the effort onto your abs during the movement. This lower back position will protect your lower back from injury whilst also allowing a bigger flexion of the upper/ mid part of the spine, resulting in a more quality abdominal contraction for the upper abs.

Whatever abdominal exercise you are performing, the breathing is performed in the same way. "Breathing out on the effort and keeping your abs tight" is a phrase that I've used for way over twenty years and to be fair, it should be totally worn out by now!

Joking aside though, if you can get the correct breathing technique, especially with abs specific exercises, you will have a flatter stomach. It works like this:

Once you are in position to perform an abs exercise, hold this position while you exhale. On exhaling, you will get to where your abs naturally engage. Once at this point, consciously take over the abs engagement and pull your stomach muscles in so your abdominals are flat.

Once here, you should be able to keep your abs in this position while breathing normally. This is what I mean when I say "keep your abs tight". During the exercise set, you can breathe out on the effort (the contraction) and breathe in on the way back to the start position.

If you are finding this hard to master at first, try simply holding and breathing normally whilst in the start position, with your abs set and ready to go. If you are a total beginner and find this hard, don't worry! You can see this as part of the progression; you will develop your abs simply by doing this exercise.

To sum this up:

- When performing lower abs exercises, make sure you get that hip tilt in, bring your knees and legs high and flex your lower spine to channel the effort onto your abdominals.
- When performing upper abs exercises, again, make sure you tilt your hips to push your lower back into the floor or bench.
- Make sure you get a good start to each set with your "abs tight".
- Keep your stomach flat throughout your set and remember to breathe correctly. Practice breathing and holding in the start position if you find this difficult at first.

Here are the variations of abdominal exercises that can target the upper, lower, or both parts of the abs.

As per the "Big 5" exercises, there are progressions you can work towards with these exercises, so try to perfect each one before moving on to the next progression. Again, these exercise descriptions and illustrations are shown in the "Exercise Descriptions" section of this book.

I've set up the core exercises slightly differently than the rest of the exercises. You will notice with the options for upper abs, lower abs and lower back, rather than having a set progression path, you will be able to identify the difficulty by beginner intermediate or advanced.

Upper abs

- Seated crunch – Beginner
- Crunches, wrist to knees – Beginner
- Crunches, fingers on temples – Intermediate
- Exercise ball crunch – Intermediate
- Crunches, feet raised – Advanced
- V sit crunch - Advanced

Lower abs

- Single knee raise – Beginner
- Double knee raise – Beginner
- Leg raise – Intermediate
- Seated knee raises – Intermediate
- Hanging knee raise – Advanced
- Hanging leg raise – Advanced

Lower back

- The stabiliser – Beginner
- Cat cow stretch – Beginner
- Double leg bridge – Intermediate
- Alternate swim – Intermediate
- Dorsal raise – Intermediate
- Superhero – Advanced
- Single leg bridge – Advanced

When deciding which abs exercises to pick for your workout routines, if you are new to this type of training, I would advise picking a beginner exercise variation of both upper, lower abs along with a beginner variation of a lower back exercise, so you should have three core exercises to work on before moving on to the intermediate variations.

Spine mobility is a good thing and will always benefit a healthy trainer with no prior injuries, provided that it is done correctly and under control. With this said though, if you are someone who suffers from back pain, it may be uncomfortable to work the abs in this way. Lower back pain is extremely common and if you are a sufferer, you may want to prioritise your recovery through strengthening and mobility of the lower back before jumping right into these abs exercises.

The lower back is a big part of your core strength and stability. And personally, I see the lower back to be as important as the abdominals. If you have strong abs but a weak lower back, you will probably suffer from back pain or at least leave yourself open to the possibility of developing lower back pain or injury at some point.

As it is with the abs, it is with the lower back muscles in that we can strengthen them up by performing all the other bodyweight exercises. Providing our exercise form is good. But there are ways to target the lower back specifically. We can do this with mobility movements and weight bearing movements.

When targeting the lower back, it's important to remember that the range of movement is limited by the mechanics of the spine. The spine does not have hinges and primary moving muscles attached to it like the arms, legs, and shoulders do. This means that by their nature, the lower back muscles are actually designed to be stabiliser muscles that work in synergy with the glutes.

So if you want to target your lower back with specific movements, it's more reasonable to think of isometric related exercises. But as the glutes are connected to the lower back muscles, we can target these with small, dynamic movements that have a direct synergy with those lower back muscles.

There are several lower back strengthening exercises in the "Exercise Descriptions" section of this book, and just like all the other exercises, there are several progressions, starting from beginner and leading to more advanced movements.

It's worth mentioning again that lower back pain is very common. Lower back pain can be avoided or corrected with the right core conditioning, so if you are free of lower back pain right now, you should definitely add some form of lower back strengthening to your workouts to keep it this way. Remember that if you have strong abs, you will want a strong lower back to balance it out, so it's wise not to neglect this area.

If you are one of the many people suffering from lower back pain, it's a good idea not to jump right into the dynamic glute/ lower back exercises right away. Instead, look to incorporate the lower back mobility exercises into your routine. This will still give you an element of lower back strengthening, but in my experience, developing good mobility is the foundation of any physical progression and is the priority of any rehabilitation effort.

Everyone is different, however, and if you are a sufferer of lower back pain, it is certainly worth visiting a physiotherapist. Find one that is well qualified and enthusiastic about their profession if you go down this route and you will not be disappointed.

Negative & Eccentric Training

Negative training or eccentric training (the same thing with several names) is a great way to improve strength, exercise form, and it can help with progression if you hit a plateau on most exercises. For example, if you are struggling to transition from an assisted variation of pull-ups to standard pull ups, negative training is an option.

Sticking with the exercise example of "Standard pull ups" and the transition from assisted to full pull ups, you may be stuck doing bodyweight rows comfortably but are finding it impossible to perform a single, standard pull up. This is certainly a common position to be in, but using negatives or eccentric training can get you past this roadblock.

To get past this hurdle, you will need a pullup bar or something to do pullups on. You can be creative here, but just make sure that your chosen pullup tool is sturdy and can hold your weight. There are plenty of ways that you can improvise, but I would highly recommend that you pick up an actual bar. These are inexpensive and easy to store, especially the bars that fit over, or between a door frame.

Once you have all the means to perform a full pullup, this is how negative or eccentric training works in furthering progression with this exercise:

Position yourself so you are at the top of the movement. To do this, it's best to use a step or chair. It is possible to jump into this position, but I wouldn't advise it as you will have more control and a better start position by stepping off a raised surface.

When getting into the start position for a negative rep, make sure this is at maximum contraction, meaning that you are at full range of movement for the exercise. With pull-ups, this means that your chin is in line with the bar. This way you will work the muscles through the whole movement and nothing will be neglected on the negative rep.

To reinforce the importance of exercise form, and indeed the start position of any negative rep it should be ingrained in your mind that working the muscles through this full range of movement is the exact reason to perform negatives and the strength at each increment of the movement matters.

With this in mind, once you are in this start position, lower yourself to the regular start position for the exercise under control, so when you are finished the rep, you are at full extension. The slower and smoother that you can do this, the better, as your muscles will be at tension through the full range of movement, challenging them at every stage.

When you are at full extension (the normal start position for standard pull ups) you have completed one rep. Have a few seconds' rest and set up for another rep. You can do this for as many times as you can until you lose your form and become fatigued.

This type of training can apply to most exercises, so can also be used if you are struggling to transition from one progression of exercise to the next.

Training with negatives can be a great way to progress, but control and form is extremely important here and this can't be overemphasised. If you are not in control of a negative and you allow your joints and ligaments to jolt and overstretch at the bottom of a movement, this can cause injury.

So if you are going to give negatives a try, it's important that you have a base amount of strength and you understand the correct form of the exercise choice fully before jumping in, therefore I would not recommend negatives for total beginners.

Isometrics

Isometric training can be used exclusively or it can run alongside other methods of resistance training. It is an excellent way to develop muscle strength and tone. Rather than just mentioning isometric training and giving examples of isometric exercises, I feel that this training method deserves more of a spotlight and a deeper explanation. If Bruce Lee put a big emphasis on isometric training, we should definitely hold it in high regard! Yes, the master of the one inch punch was into this type of training.

So we know that isometric training means:

"Bodyweight exercise that has a static form to strengthen varying muscle groups,"

But how do you put this into practice? Where does it fit in to your training and how can you get the most out of it?

There are three different ways to train with isometrics that I would like to cover, so let's jump in.

Flexing your muscles.

At the beginning of the training for my first bodybuilding show, I had no interest in isometric training, I just lifted heavy weights to pump up those muscles, each rep of each exercise was about two seconds up and two seconds down and I could lift some heavy weights in this way.

I had been training like this, seriously for about seven years, before deciding to actually commit and sign up for a bodybuilding show. Luckily for me, the guy who ran the gym I used at the time was a veteran bodybuilder who had competed many times before and had a whole bunch of winner trophies on his shelf, he was a personal trainer and really knew his stuff, and he really took an interest in anyone who decided to compete in a show. He created our diet plans, helped us with training if we needed it, he gave us discounted protein shakes; he took care of organising the competition registration, so all we had to do was train and eat.

He also taught us how to pose on stage. Anyone who has not been involved in bodybuilding competition may see the posing side of bodybuilding as an ego thing. But this is far from reality. You could have the best physique in the world, but if you can't show it to the judges when you are on stage, you may not get very far in the competition.

After most training sessions, my coach would grab me and the two other guys that where going for the same competition and he would take us through a bunch of poses, front double bicep, side chest, abs and quads, quarter turns to name a few. This was exhausting!

It was really tough for us as we were not used to holding these poses. We had not trained in this way before. This was isometric training.

In the first few weeks, we would hold some poses for only a few seconds before starting to shake. Holding a pose meant that you slowly moved into the position, and once there, you would hold at maximum muscle contraction. So a "front double bicep pose" would see us standing front on, knees slightly bent, arms up and tensed to show off the biceps. We aimed to hold each pose for at least 30 seconds.

Although there are poses with names that are supposed to show specific muscle groups like the "double bicep", in a competition, you are always judged on your whole body, so keeping your abs and legs tensed is also a must.

Keeping your full body under tension for periods of time is hard work. It takes a lot of energy and muscular stamina, but if you do this regularly, your body will adapt and become stronger, develop more stamina and the muscles will become more defined and solid.

Twenty weeks into our posing sessions, we could hold each pose for as long as we needed to. There was no shaking of tired muscles and it became more comfortable to do this. I believe that these posing sessions had a big impact on my overall muscular definition, giving me a leaner, more ripped look than I would have had if I'd not have taken it as seriously.

Tensing or flexing your muscles under their own tension is certainly a good introduction to using isometrics, so have a go at singling out each muscle group and tensing them. You can even do this sitting down. Try tensing and holding your quads and hamstrings, your biceps, your glutes or your pecs. This action will not only engage these muscles, but as you get used to singling out these muscle groups, it will also allow you to perform better during other resistance training.

Flexing with your own resistance.

Building on this idea of flexing your muscle groups under their own tension, you can add resistance to this by using other body parts to push or pull against. For example, you could perform a static bicep curl but rather than just flexing the muscle, you could attempt to perform a full bicep curl but have your other arm hold it back by clasping your hands together.

This can be done in several ways for different muscle groups. If you want to add this into your training or give it a go, think about the mechanics of each muscle group you want to work and perform that movement while adding enough resistance to make the exercise static.

Your own bodyweight can also count as your own resistance. If you hold yourself in any variation of a push up or pull up, you are performing an isometric exercise under your own resistance.

Immovable objects

Isometric training using immovable objects is probably the most used and arguably the most effective.

To do this, you will need some immovable objects such as solid walls, fixed posts, doorways, or you can actually buy exercise kit that is made specifically for this.

Imagine performing a bicep curl with a solid bar that was fixed in position, or doing a pec fly, but instead of using dumbbells or a machine, you use a fixed length of rope, squats using a bar permanently fixed at chest height, deadlift from a bar on a short chain that's fixed into the floor, or even trying to push a wall down.

There are a few things to remember when training like this. Although the movements can be the same or very similar to movements you would do with dumbbells and barbells in the gym, you need to consider the amount of force you use, the speed at which you use it and the time per rep.

The force

When using force, ideally, you should aim for 60% of your max effort as a beginner, building this up to 100% as you progress. This will ensure you are challenging your muscles enough for them to develop whilst also protecting and prepping your joints and tendons for this type of exercise.

The speed

It's not great to start an isometric rep right at your maximum effort of force, even if you are a beginner and you are only going to be pushing 60% effort. If you go from 0% to 60% or even 100% immediately, you are putting yourself at risk of injury, injury that can easily be avoided.

You only need to take the first 2 to 3 seconds after you are in position to slowly build up to your target effort. At the end of the isometric rep, you should also do this in reverse. Don't just immediately relax, slowly wind down the force over 2 or 3 seconds. This will give your muscles and joints time to adjust, along with giving you the extra control and stability for solid muscular development.

The time

When training with isometrics, a big factor and measure of progress is the time spent under tension. A good range to work in is 6 to 12 second holds.

With an isometric bicep curl, for example, we may perform holds of 8 seconds with a 60% force. When this becomes less challenging over time, we can look at increasing the time on the hold, the amount of force on the hold, or both of these factors. This is how progression works with isometric training.

A walkthrough

Sticking with the example of an isometric bicep curl, this is a walkthrough of one "rep" or one "hold" for clarity.

Get yourself into the start position for a bicep curl gripping the static bar or whatever immovable object you are using for this exercise and take a grip. At this point, you are just concentrating on your position and form applying no pressure.

At the start of the rep, slowly and under control, over the first 2 or 3 seconds of your hold, apply force smoothly until you reach your target workload. If you are a beginner, look for around 60% of your max effort.

Once at your target workload, hold until you reach your target time and then over 2 or 3 seconds, slowly and smoothly release the tension. Remember to keep your breathing continuous and controlled throughout the rep.

Three ranges of isometrics

The last thing I would like to mention on isometric training is the range of position for exercise choices.

When performing traditional exercises with dumbbells, barbells and calisthenics, each rep of an exercise has a range of movement. Keeping good exercise form and working your muscles through the full range of movement is the way to go if you want to get the most out of the exercise.

When using isometric exercises, however, we can only set one range of movement for each rep. The most common approach is to set the range at the mid-point of the exercise. But if you want to work isometrics through a full range of movement, you can do this by working at full extension, mid-range and maximum contraction.

We've used bicep curls as the example in the rest of this chapter, so let's stick with it for an example of a full range isometric workout. You can change the range on any type of isometric, whether this is flexing, flexing under your own tension or using immovable objects, the principal is the same.

Here's a description with illustrations of bicep curls at the different ranges mentioned.

Full extension

Full extension is the point at which the muscles are at their most extended, or they are at their most "stretched". With bicep curls, this is when the arm is straight and the elbow is close to locking out. An important take away here is when working at full extension with exercise of this nature, take the term "full extension" to mean "just before joint lock out".

Mid-range

The mid-range is the mid-point between full extension and maximum contraction. As mentioned, this is the most popular position to work in with isometrics. The logic is that the mid-range will give the most stability and balance between max contraction and full extension.

Maximum contraction

Maximum contraction is the point at which the muscle is at its shortest. If you are familiar with any of my other fitness books that have exercise descriptions inside, I use the term "top of movement" to describe this.

Isometrics with bodyweight training

You can take most, if not all, the bodyweight exercises mentioned in this book and use them for isometric training. When creating your own routine using the program cards provided, there is a column marked "time". So if you want to use the exercise "standard dips" as an isomeric exercise, for example, you can decide on the amount of sets (this will be how many times you will perform the exercise) and then decide on the time that you aim to hold the isometric movement for. This can be measured in seconds or even minutes, depending on how "Bruce Lee" you are. ☺

When it comes to upgrading your exercise card, you can aim for a longer time, increase the reps or both to make this more challenging and progress with your isometric holds.

Exercise Equipment?

The draw to bodyweight training for many people is the fact that to do it effectively, you don't need a gym membership, and you can actually use your bodyweight as the workload.

While this is true, you can greatly enhance your training, upgrade your exercise choices, hit muscle groups from different angles, increase range of motion and add another dimension to your workouts with a few pieces of exercise equipment designed for bodyweight exercise movements.

If you are totally new to bodyweight training, explore the possibilities without equipment as a starting point. There is a lot to learn, not only exercise choices and form, but you will also be able to identify your strengths and weaknesses.

As a beginner, there is a lot more scope for development and progression without extra equipment, too, as your body will probably be challenged enough with the basics to develop strength and muscle at this point.

If you are not ready to invest in any training equipment just yet, for whatever reason, there are still plenty of ways to improvise. Most homes have chairs that can be used for dips, assisted squats, incline pushups and such. There are plenty of walls, door frames, kitchen corner surfaces and things like loft hatches to get creative with.

Most public children's play areas have more than one option to perform bodyweight exercises from, although this is not ideal for several reasons, it's still a viable option. It's becoming increasingly popular however, for local councils and communities to build "outdoor gyms" that are specifically designed for this type of training and these have many similarities to that of a kid's play area, so if you are lucky enough to have access to one of these, this is a very good option.

Improvising with every day, household furniture is fine for the short term, but I would recommend investing in a few pieces of exercise equipment that are specifically designed for this type of exercise.

With kit that's made for the job, you will have a better experience as you will be able to concentrate on form, body positioning and performance that bit more. These pieces of exercise equipment are also pretty easy to store.

Here are the pieces of equipment that I suggest you invest in.

Dip bars

Dip bars are pretty versatile as you can use them for more than just dips. As well as dips, they can also be used for rows, incline push ups, assisted squats and such. If you are looking to move onto more advanced exercises like L sits, planch and other isometric exercises, dips bars will be even more useful to you.

There are several types of dip bars that also have a broad price range. Some of these bars are part of a bigger piece of kit, which will obviously require you to have a lot more room if you choose one of these. Some are made as a frame rather than individual bars and so on. I have a set of dip bars that are individual so they can be spaced differently if needed and this is also better for storage.

When it comes to your choice, as long as the bars are sturdy and high enough for you to do full dips on, this is all that really matters when it comes to the exercise, but space and storage when these bars are not in use is definitely worth a thought.

Paralletts or push up bars

To the new trainer, these are not really an essential piece of kit. I say this because when considering the "big 5" exercises, you can get by without them. They are, however, excellent for progression training. When considering the use of push up bars and paralletts bars with the exercises push ups and shoulder press, you can add an extra dimension in the form of a bigger range of movement.

The function of paralletts and push up bars are to raise the floor to give you extra clearance for a bigger movement. With this in mind, there are some really easy substitutes for these pieces of kit. You could use a couple of bricks, for example. But the big benefit with investing in a quality, purpose made training equipment of this nature is that you will get the stability and ergonomics to give you a much better training experience than you might have if you decided to improvise.

Pull up bars

Pull up bars are another piece of kit that have a wide variation of style, quality and price. Again, these are widely available. A good option for space saving is a pull up bard that fits in a door frame. You can pick up some good quality pull up bars in this category, but you can also pick up some horrible ones. I prefer the bars that fit through the door, hook onto the top frame and are supported both sides of the door.

These bars allow you to work outside the actual door frame, giving you more room and often come with handles for regular pull ups and handles for an inverse grip, which gives a lot more versatility.

Exercises ball

This is a piece of exercise kit that does take up a lot of space, but because it's basically an inflatable, it can be deflated and stored fairly easily. If you are tight on space, however, and decide to only inflate the ball when you are going to work out, it becomes a big inconvenience.

If you have the space, the pros far outweigh the cons. You can use an exercise ball for exercises variations that require stability, such as hack squats. You can use it as a bench for certain exercises and I have even used an exercise ball as my office chair for a time in the past. This is not an essential piece of kit for bodyweight workouts, but if you have the space, it's definitely worth a consideration. I've added a great abs exercise using an exercise ball in to the exercise descriptions for those who have one of these to try.

Bench

Exercise benches are not essential, but if you have the room and finances, they can be very useful. A quality exercise bench will give you stability with resistance training and although you can use a regular chair for things like "bench squats" or "incline push ups", a bench will give you extra stability and a better experience. With that said, not all of us have the room for a bench, but if you do, it's worth a consideration.

Exercise bands

Whenever anyone shows interest in fitness training of any kind, especially if this is resistance based and the goal is to "lose weight and tone up", exercise bands are an excellent piece of kit to have. If you know what to do with exercise bands, you technically have a small gym that fits into a bag. There are times when you can integrate exercise bands into your bodyweight training (we will cover some examples of this in the exercise descriptions section). These are not essential for bodyweight training but are very useful to have around.

To sum this up, all you really need is a good quality pull-up bar and a set of dip bars that suit your storage space. You can get by without these, but the experience will not be as good and you will have to get creative.

The Warm Up

There is some controversy over pre workout warmups. Some say there is no need to do any warm up, and some say that warmups are vital. The truth is that it's down to the individual to decide. The more experience that an individual has with training and exercise, the better qualified they are to decide whether the workout ahead of them warrants a warmup, and to what degree.

I believe that before doing resistance training of any kind, you should always complete a warm up to some extent. This warmup could simply be localised to the muscle group being trained. An example of this is that if you were going to focus on improving your pullups in a training session, you would complete a few light sets of incline rows to stimulate the back and trap muscles along with the mobility in the shoulder joints.

After this kind of warmup, your muscles you were going to be using for your pullups would be warm and have increased elasticity and the shoulder joints would also have been stimulated and ready for a bigger workload.

All too often, injuries are caused because muscles are trained when they are cold. With bodyweight training and calisthenics, pre training warmups to reduce the risk of injury are arguably the main reason to indeed complete a warmup.

A warm up before exercise does not have to be complicated or take up too much time. If you approach every workout with a few small pieces of biological knowledge, you will drastically reduce the chance of injury. You may even have a much more efficient workout.

The first basic principle for a warmup is to increase your core body temperature. To do this, all you have to do is to get moving. You could go for a quick jog, run up a few flights of stairs, jump some rope, jog on the spot, anything that increases your heart rate.

The second basic principle is stretching and mobility. Once you have an elevated heart rate and your blood is flowing through your muscles, you can now work on mobility. Mobility can be stretching muscle groups and moving joints through their full range of motion.

So if you are going to be working with a full-body workout session, you might choose to elevate your heart rate by going for a quick jog and immediately afterwards, work on the mobility of each muscle group and body part before getting into the workout.

The detail of stretching and mobility leads to a sizeable chunk of information that detracts from this guide, but I feel it is important to give a nod to the subject.

The bottom line is that performing an intense workout on a body that's not primed for the workload can lead to injury. If you want to minimise the risk of injury, you should get your heart rate up, blood flowing, and move your joins through their range of motion before getting stuck into the workout.

Your Personalised Training Plan

If you are serious about training and want results of any kind, you should have a plan. Whether this is bodyweight and calisthenics, bodybuilding or running, you should always create a plan or routine before getting started.

The idea of planning and creating a routine is something that I push into every fitness guide that I have written. Having a good plan that's progressive will challenge your current ability, aligns with your goals and is tied to some form of timescale will give you all the essential elements for success and true progression.

It's really common for a new trainer to decide that they want to achieve a specific fitness goal and set out on the actual physical part of this journey on an ad hoc basis with no proper plan. Inevitably, this will lead to zero progression and zero results. Sounds harsh, but this is very true.

If a small amount of time is invested into creating a fitness plan from the beginning that suited the trainer, there is a much better chance that progression will be made and results will be earned.

Learning how to create your own exercise routine is a very valuable skill, especially if you want to take this seriously. Learning how to upgrade your plan is also something that will keep you progressing and in this section, we will look at how to go about this, so you can effectively become your own personal trainer.

The bodyweight training plans that are about to be created in this chapter can be used directly by you if they fit your spec, but you can also change up and tweak things here and there to suit you better. If this is nowhere near your needs, you can simply start your own from scratch.

This part of the book will take you through my process of creating a personalised bodyweight training routine in a step-by-step process you can follow along with.

Who is this for?

The first thing to determine is who this routine is for. Even if you are creating this routine for yourself, ask this question. If the routine you create is too difficult and is beyond the scope of your abilities, it won't be effective. On the other side of the coin, if it's too easy and doesn't challenge you enough, again, it won't be effective.

In this example, I'm going to be creating an exercise routine for a guy called Jimmy thirty years old, has no prior experience in fitness and works an office job that offers very little in the way of physical labour. Jimmy has decided that he wants to get into shape by using a bodyweight routine.

Jimmy is 5 foot and 9 inches tall with an average build, but is around the 30 per cent mark when it comes to body fat. If you were not a fitness professional, you could describe Jimmy as "an average thirty-year-old who is fairly out of shape". Fair play to Jimmy, though. He wants to get in shape, so let's do it!

We will fill in the simple exercise cards that I have designed to run alongside this guide. If you are reading the paperback version, you will find a bunch of blank exercise cards at the back of this book that you can photocopy or just straight up write on.

If you are reading the eBook version, please feel free to contact me via one of my social media channels or email and I'll be more than happy to send you over a PDF copy of the blank card so you have limitless access.

The exercises

We know that the big 5 is our bread and butter training, so this is where we will start. As Jimmy has no prior experience in fitness, it is very sensible to start on the first progressions of these exercises.

So the exercise choices from the big 5 that we will start the creation of Jimmy's routine with are:

- Standing push ups
- Incline rows
- Assisted dips
- Standing incline press
- Assisted squats

BODYWEIGHT TRAINING			

ROUTINE #	1		

EXERCISE	SETS	REPS	TIME
Standing push ups			
Incline Rows			
Assisted Dips			
Standing incline Press			
Assisted Squats			

WEEKS	MON	TUE	WED	THURS	FRI	SAT	SUN
1							
2							
3							
4							
5							

As Jimmy is a total beginner, we also want him to develop a strong core so we will add both an upper, lower abs exercise along with a lower back stretch.

The upper and lower abs exercises will be chosen from the beginner progressions list as Jimmy will need to build up his abdominal strength alongside his big 5 movements and again, as Jimmy is a beginner, this is a sensible place to start. I have also added a lower back exercise as a stretch to Jimmy's routine. The reason for this is to ensure that Jimmy is working on mobility of the lower back as a priority.

When following any resistance routine that incorporates abdominal work, I always suggest that these exercises are tagged on to the end of the session. My reason for this is that abs and core muscles are being engaged and used as stabilisers and synergists in every other exercise, so it makes sense to keep them fresh for this important role. When you isolate the core muscles and put them through their paces, this will lead to fatigue and they have potential to be less effective as stabilisers after this.

This is especially important for beginners. With this said, there are slight exceptions to this rule with things like circuit training, but I do not recommend training methods like circuit training for the total beginner.

So the abs and core exercises for Jimmy are:

- Crunches, wrists to knees (for upper abs)
- Lying knee raises (for lower abs)
- Cat cow (lower back mobility)

BODYWEIGHT TRAINING & CALISTHENICS

BODYWEIGHT TRAINING			

ROUTINE #	1		

EXERCISE	SETS	REPS	TIME
Standing push ups			
Incline Rows			
Assisted Dips			
Standing incline Press			
Assisted Squats			
Crunches, Wrists to knees			
Lying knee raise, single leg			
Cat cow			

WEEKS	MON	TUE	WED	THURS	FRI	SAT	SUN
1							
2							
3							
4							
5							

The workload

With dynamic resistance exercises (isotonic movements), meaning the muscles contract and then lengthen, the measure of "sets and reps" is the way to go if you are looking for full muscular development. A "rep" is a "repetition" of an exercise and a set is the amount of times you will do a "set" number of "reps".

The number of sets and reps can have a big range, depending on your goals and ability. As Jimmy is a beginner, we will choose to keep it modest with a pattern of 2 sets of 10 reps for all exercises bar one.

Because Jimmy is going to be working with the early exercise progressions, he should find this range doable. These exercises have less resistance than the later variations to also make them fit nicely into this pattern and ability level.

The exception to these sets and reps range is the lower back stretch. I have chosen 2 sets of 6 reps and have utilised the "time" column. The reason for this is that the exercise "cat cow" is a double movement and a hold as well as a rep. There is a start position, a top of movement for the back arch (flexion of the spine) and then an extension of the spine for the second position. For both the flexion and extension of the spine, Jimmy will hold the position for 3 seconds.

BODYWEIGHT TRAINING & CALISTHENICS

BODYWEIGHT TRAINING			

ROUTINE #	1		

EXERCISE	SETS	REPS	TIME
Standing push ups	2	10	-----
Incline Rows	2	10	-----
Assisted Dips	2	10	-----
Standing incline Press	2	10	-----
Assisted Squats	2	10	-----
Crunches, Wrists to knees	2	10	-----
Lying knee raise, single leg	2	10	-----
Cat cow	2	6	3 secs

WEEKS	MON	TUE	WED	THURS	FRI	SAT	SUN
1							
2							
3							
4							
5							

The time scale

There are two parts to the timescale of an exercise routine; how long you stick to this routine for (this is going to be measured in weeks) and how often you will follow the routine (this is going to be measured in days per week).

As this is a beginner routine that's tailored to Jimmy, I would advise that he completes this work out three times per week on non-consecutive days to start with. Having at least one day's break between workouts will give his body chance to recover and prepare for the next session. Rest and recovery play a big part in fitness and progression. And for Jimmy, this routine is challenging his body more than his is used to.

The same routine can be done for varying lengths of time. Depending on your ability and your goal, the same routine can be followed anywhere from one week to twelve weeks. In some cases, the same routine can run without an end date. From my experience, the great thing about beginners is that they will develop and progress a lot quicker than more practiced trainers. I believe this is because once someone's natural potential has been unlocked and reached; they will have the extra challenge of getting through training plateaus, which sometimes means a total rethink of exercise choices, methods, workload and such.

For Jimmy's first exercise routine, I am going to set his routine to be completed for four weeks to start with. Four weeks is a good benchmark for establishing new habits and if Jimmy is consistent with his training slots in this time, he should definitely see an improvement in his strength and ability to perform the exercises. He may even see significant development in as little as two weeks.

So Jimmy's exercise card will be marked with a check against the days he will train that correspond with the week in the table at the bottom of the card.

BODYWEIGHT TRAINING			

ROUTINE #	1		

EXERCISE	SETS	REPS	TIME
Standing push ups	2	10	-----
Incline Rows	2	10	-----
Assisted Dips	2	10	-----
Standing incline Press	2	10	-----
Assisted Squats	2	10	-----
Crunches, Wrists to knees	2	10	-----
Lying knee raise, single leg	2	10	-----
Cat cow	2	6	3 secs

WEEKS	MON	TUE	WED	THURS	FRI	SAT	SUN
1	*		*		*		
2	*		*		*		
3	*		*		*		
4	*		*		*		
5							

Reassess & progress

This is the last part of following a fitness routine. Once you have been working out in the same way for a certain amount of time, you will become used to the training. This is a great thing! It means the exercises that you have been doing will be easier, you will struggle less in your workouts. What's actually happening is that you are getting stronger, your muscles are developing and adapting to the workload. When this happens, it's time to step it up and become even better.

Your first assessment of your new program should be during your early workouts in your first week. Ask yourself these questions on each exercise:

- Is my form perfect for this exercise?

This is always your priority. If your exercise form is not great, you will not only be potentially diluting the effect of the movement, but you could train yourself into a bad posture and opening yourself up to injury. So exercise form is your priority. If you think you can improve on your form of an exercise, work on this before anything else.

- Is this exercise too easy or too hard for me?

If your form is great but the exercise is too easy, you can simply switch it out for an upgrade at any point. Just update your exercise card. The sooner you can start challenging yourself and working with upgraded exercises, the quicker you will progress. If you have been over ambitious with a certain exercise choice, this is no problem. Again, just upgrade your program card and work from one of the earlier progressions of that exercise. It's far more valuable to be challenging yourself with an earlier progression with good exercise form than struggling to finish a set of a more advanced variation of that move.

- Can I stay consistent with this time frame?

Staying consistent is a big deal for fitness progression, and you can make it easier for yourself by planning your training sessions around your life. Does the training schedule that you have set out for yourself allow you to actually get your sessions completed? If not, you can reassess week by week if you need to, so make sure you can fit them in on every day of every week that you mark down.

Once you have completed your first program card according to your original time frame, it's time to make a new one for your next progression! If you struggled through your first program and you are still being challenged in your workouts, there is no issue in repeating the exact program again. If you are still being challenged, you are still benefiting.

Maybe some exercises are becoming easy, but some are not. In this situation, you can simply add upgrades to the ones that you are doing well on. Look to try out the next progression of the exercises that you are more comfortable. Sometimes, you may skip a progression and move right from a beginner onto an advanced exercise. But always remember your exercise form.

There are lots of other variables that you can change on your upgraded programs. Think about:

- Increasing the sets, reps or time of an exercise
- Adding more exercises
- Adding more than one variation of the same exercise
- Adding more training days
- Targeting weak muscle groups with multiple exercises
- Creating a "split training routine" (two different programs, A and B)
- Changing the training method; circuit training, superset training, etc.

It's important to remember that everyone is different and everyone progresses at a different pace, but as long as you are challenging yourself, continue looking to progress and improve, stay consistent with your training, you will be rewarded.

In the next section, there are more examples of exercise routines. If you feel that these align with your goals and abilities, go ahead and use them as they are. But remember that there are plenty of blank cards at the back of the book for you to experiment with and create something that will suit you more directly.

If you are going to create your own routine, have a good look at all the exercises and their progressions in the "exercise descriptions" section for inspiration.

Whether you are on the isometric team, the calisthenics team or a bit of both, being creative, having a goal, and having fun is a major part of bodyweight training. Learning a new skill or talent is empowering and it can change your whole life positively. So enjoy the journey of creating your routine and seeing yourself improve in strength, shape and ability from week to week.

Exercise Routines

In the previous chapter, we used Jimmy as an example of a beginner to create an exercise routine. This finished exercise routine can serve as an example for other beginners, so if you are a beginner too, and have no problems with the exercise choices that we made for Jimmy, go ahead and use this beginner routine as it is. Once you have trained in this way for a short while, you will know whether you need to tweak anything.

In this chapter, I've set up a few exercise routines of different ability levels that you can use straight out of the book or take inspiration from if you are going to create your own.

Have a look through and see if there are any that might suit you as they are. There might be parts of a beginner routine that suit you and there might be other parts from more advanced routines that suit you, too. If this is the case, use one of the blank program cards at the back and fill it in merging the parts that you want. This way, you have something of your own to follow.

With each of the following exercise routines, there is a brief explanation and some notes that I considered when creating them. This may also give you some ideas and inspiration in terms of possibilities and what to think about in your own creation.

JAMES ATKINSON

Beginner routines

BODYWEIGHT TRAINING			

ROUTINE #	1		

EXERCISE	SETS	REPS	TIME
Standing push ups	2	10	- - - - -
Incline Rows	2	10	- - - - -
Assisted Dips	2	10	- - - - -
Standing incline Press	2	10	- - - - -
Assisted Squats	2	10	- - - - -
Crunches, Wrists to knees	2	10	- - - - -
Lying knee raise, single leg	2	10	- - - - -
Cat cow	2	6	3 secs

WEEKS	MON	TUE	WED	THURS	FRI	SAT	SUN
1	*		*		*		
2	*		*		*		
3	*		*		*		
4	*		*		*		
5							

** For clarity, this is Jimmy's card that we put together in the previous chapter.

BODYWEIGHT TRAINING			

ROUTINE #	1		

EXERCISE	SETS	REPS	TIME
Standing push ups	3	10	- - - - -
Incline push ups	2	10	- - - - -
Engage and hang	5	10	5 secs
Incline rows	3	10	- - - - -
Assisted Squats	3	10	- - - - -
Crunches, Wrists to knees	3	10	- - - - -
Lying knee raise, single leg	3	10	- - - - -
The stabiliser	3	6	3 secs

WEEKS	MON	TUE	WED	THURS	FRI	SAT	SUN
1	*		*		*		
2	*		*		*		
3	*		*		*		
4	*		*		*		
5							

Notes on this beginner routine

This is a beginner routine that is designed for someone whose goals are to build upper body strength with more of a focus on pull up progression.

The first 4 exercises are designed to build shoulder strength and prepare for pull up progression. The sets and reps are standard bar only 2 exercises. Incline push ups can be classed as an intermediate level exercise, so the sets and lower.

Exercises that are timed can be tested and re assessed once they have been practiced in the first workout. Some of these times may be ambitious and individual ability will vary a lot from person to person, but this is easy to tweak once practiced.

Intermediate routines

BODYWEIGHT TRAINING

ROUTINE #	1	

EXERCISE	SETS	REPS	TIME
Incline Push ups	3	10	-----
Negative Pull ups	3	6	-----
Seated dips	3	10	----
Pike Press	3	10	-----
Seat Squats	3	10	------
Crunches, fingers on temples	3	10	-----
Double knee raise	3	10	-----
The stabiliser	3	6	3 secs

WEEKS	MON	TUE	WED	THURS	FRI	SAT	SUN
1	*		*		*		
2	*		*		*		
3	*		*		*		
4	*		*		*		
5							

Notes on this intermediate routine

This routine could be used as an introduction for someone who already has a base level of strength and fitness. It can also be used as an upgrade to one of the beginner programs.

We are looking at 3 sets of 10 reps as standard, bar the negative pull ups and the stabiliser. These can be tweaked to suite based on the individuals' ability. At this level, to give an extra challenge, the sets of some exercises could be increased to 4 and the reps could be increased to 12 on exercises that are less challenging.

BODYWEIGHT TRAINING			

ROUTINE #			

EXERCISE	SETS	REPS	TIME
Standard Push ups	3	12	-----
Engage and hang	4	1	8 secs
Negative pull ups	6	10	----
Seated dips	3	12	-----
Pike press	3	12	-----
Bodyweight squats	3	12	-----
Crunches., Fingers on temples	3	12	-----
Seated knee raise	3	12	-----
Double leg bridge	3	12	-----

WEEKS	MON	TUE	WED	THURS	FRI	SAT	SUN
1	*		*		*		*
2	*		*		*		*
3	*		*		*		*
4	*		*		*		*
5							

Notes on this intermediate routine

The standard of 3 sets of 12 reps is taken with this routine apart from the "engage and hang" and "negative pull ups" exercises, as they are slightly different forms of exercise. If you use isometrics, such as the "engage and hang", remember that the time spent on the set will have a big bearing on the difficulty of that set, so be sure to adjust according to your ability.

Another difference to this training routine is that there is an extra training day added. Until you are a more advanced trainer, it's advisable not to train in this way every day, as you will need more time to recover. Once you are more conditioned, you can start training daily and switch to more advanced routines like "split training".

A more advanced training routine

This routine is a "2 day split". This means that we are working the full body over 2 different training sessions on different days. It's a more advanced way of training, but is great for planning a more intense workout on each muscle group. Take a look at the next two program cards and check out the notes for clarity.

BODYWEIGHT TRAINING & CALISTHENICS

BODYWEIGHT TRAINING			
ROUTINE #		2 day split - routine A	
EXERCISE	**SETS**	**REPS**	**TIME**
Standard Push ups	4	12	- - - - -
Push ups with bars	4	12	- - - - -
Standard pull ups	4	RF	- - - -
Negative pull ups	12	1	- - - - -
Pike press	4	12	- - - - -
Elevated pike press	4	RF	- - - - -

WEEKS	MON	TUE	WED	THURS	FRI	SAT	SUN
1	*			*			
2	*			*			
3	*			*			
4	*			*			
5	*			*			

BODYWEIGHT TRAINING			

ROUTINE #		2 day split - routine B		

EXERCISE	SETS	REPS	TIME
Bodyweight squats	4	15	- - - - -
Elevated pistol squats	4	12	- - - - -
Standard dips	4	RF	- - - -
Standard dips isometric hold	12	1	8 secs
Crunches feet raised	4	RF	- - - - -
Seated knee raise	4	RF	- - - - -

WEEKS	MON	TUE	WED	THURS	FRI	SAT	SUN
1		*			*		
2		*			*		
3		*			*		
4		*			*		
5		*			*		

Notes on this 2 day split routine

There are two routines in this split, a "workout A" and a "workout B". The "workout A" focuses on chest, back and shoulder exercises using push ups, pull ups and shoulder press exercise variations.

The "workout B" focuses on legs, triceps and abdominals using squats, dips and abs, exercise variations.

The next thing that makes this a 2 day split is the days that we are working out on. You will see that for "workout A" we are working out with this routine on Mondays and Thursdays. "Workout B" is done on Tuesdays and Fridays, so we are doing a total of 4 workouts each week, but with a higher intensity on each muscle group and exercise.

The last thing to note here is that for some exercises in the "reps" column, instead of a number, there is an "RF". This means "reasonable failure". Pushing yourself to reasonable failure on the more advanced variations of an exercise is an excellent way to progress, especially if you have pre exhausted the muscle group beforehand with a less advanced variation of that exercise.

Reasonable failure is to complete as many reps of an exercise as you can before your form deteriorates. If you try this, it's really important to learn to recognise when your exercise form is suffering due to fatigue. It's ok to try 1 or 2 reps at the point of fatigue, but lots of "cheat reps" will only really help to strengthen your ego, not your muscles. ☺

Section 2

Introduction to section 2

Here you will find the range of exercise choices with all the necessary progressions. There are at least two illustrations of each exercise that show the starting position and end position of each movement. These illustrations also show correct posture, form and have written descriptions that detail how to perform the exercise correctly.

Posture and exercise form, during exercise, is extremely important, so please have this at the forefront of your mind when practicing and performing all exercises.

Along with the illustration of each exercise, there is a description. If you are new to a certain movement, it's best to have a go at the exercises and make sure you can perform it correctly before getting into the actual workouts.

If you are creating your own exercise routine, there are some blank exercise cards for you to fill in at the back of the book.

The Exercises

Push Ups Progression

The push up is a compound exercise that utilises the chest muscles as the primary muscle group. Because this is a compound movement, the push up also uses the triceps and deltoids too. A point to note about push ups is that the bigger the incline that you use, the more the shoulders will take the workload.

As the shoulders and chest work together through this movement, there is a crossover with progression exercises. An example of a cross over exercise is the standing incline press. We can use the standing incline press as a progression for both shoulder press and push ups.

When using the standing incline press as a progression for push ups, it's beneficial to make a conscious effort to focus the work down onto your chest muscles. A tip to help with this is to keep your elbows low and drawn in slightly throughout the movement.

1st progression - Standing push ups

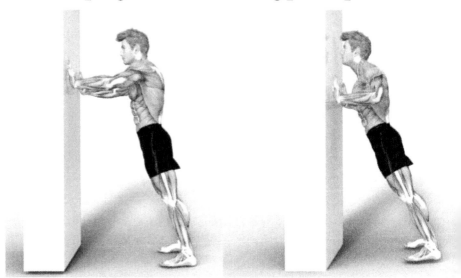

Start position

- Find a solid, upright surface to work with. A straight wall is ideal.
- Position your hands on the wall so your arms are parallel to the floor and in line with your mid chest.
- Make sure your hands are spaced so that your thumbs are in line with your outer shoulder.
- Take a step backwards so that you are taking the weight of your body.
- Keep your back flat, abs engaged and look forward.

Movement

- As you inhale, bend your arms by lowering your body towards the wall until your nose almost touches the surface.
- Your elbows should flare out only slightly.
- Once at the top of the movement, exhale as you return to the start position. This is one rep.

Extra info

Lowering yourself until your nose touches the surface will serve as a good gauge for maximum range of movement and will help you keep your back straight. Remember that the further you step back while setting up your position, the more challenging it will be, but the more of an incline that you create here will put a bigger workload on the shoulders and may take from the chest, so there is a fine line.

2nd progression – Incline push ups

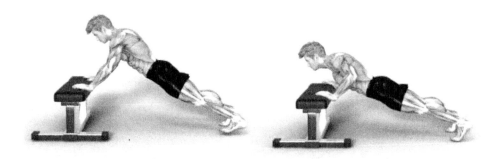

Start position

- Pick a solid surface, bench, chair, exercise step, etc.
- Position yourself over the working surface with your hands just past shoulder width apart.
- Arms straight, but elbows slightly bent.
- Your abs should be engaged and your back flat. Looking forward will help to keep this alignment.

Movement

- Lower yourself under control by bending at the elbows
- Keep your back flat and abs engaged
- Your elbows should not flare out too much to keep the workload on the chest muscles
- Breathe in on the way down and exhale when returning to the start position

Extra info

Incline push ups can be used as a progression on the path to full push-ups, and for a progression when working towards shoulder press too. When using this exercise to work towards full push-ups, you can add smaller increments of progression by reducing the height of the working surface.

The higher the working surface, the less challenge this exercise will be and vice versa.

3rd progression - Standard push ups

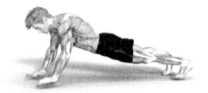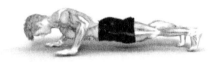

Start position

- Position yourself over the working surface with your hands just past shoulder width apart.
- Arms straight, but elbows slightly bent.
- Your abs should be engaged and your back flat. Looking forward will help to keep this alignment.

Movement

- Lower yourself under control by bending at the elbows
- Keep your back flat and abs engaged
- Your elbows should not flare out too much to keep the workload on the chest muscles
- Breathe in on the way down and exhale when returning to the start position

Extra info

Always be aware of fatigue with this exercise. Be conscious of keeping a straight back, don't let your head drop and be mindful not to let your hips sag or your back arch. Don't let your elbows flare out too much and be sure that the main workload is going through your chest muscles.

4th progression – Push ups with bars

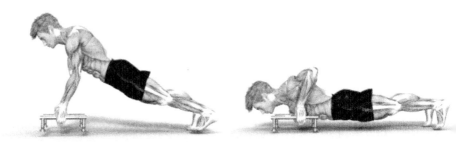

Start position

- Position your paralletts bars over the working surface so your hands are just past shoulder width apart. The bars should be parallel to each other and inline.
- Arms straight, but elbows slightly bent.
- Your abs should be engaged and your back flat. Looking forward will help to keep this alignment.

Movement

- Lower yourself under control by bending at the elbows.
- Keep your back flat and abs engaged.
- Your elbows should not flare out too much to keep the workload on the chest muscles.
- Lower yourself to where you feel the stretch.
- Breathe in on the way down and exhale when returning to the start position.
- As you perform the push up, the bars should not move.

Extra info

This is considered an advanced exercise. Be careful not to overstretch. This is possible ass some bars might be higher than others and everyone is different when it comes to mobility. A bigger range of movement is good, but if you struggle to reach the position that you would like, take it slowly and work up to it over several sessions.

If you do not have paralletts bars, you can use other solid objects to create elevated platforms for your hands. Make sure these are strong and will not slip in the middle of the exercise.

Pullups Progression

Pullups are a compound exercise that utilise the back muscles as the main working muscle group. As this is a compound exercise, performing pullups will also stimulate the biceps, trapezius and rhomboid muscles.

Many people find Pullups to be one of the most difficult exercises for to master, but with the correct progression path, it can be done. Developing the muscles of the back and biceps through other bodyweight exercises and performing negatives and isometric hangs on a pull up bar can help to speed this process along.

1st progression – Incline rows

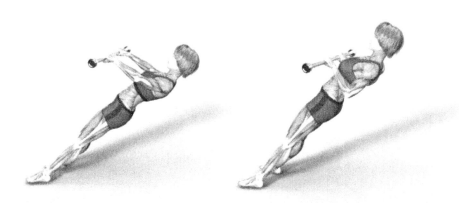

Start position

- You will need a horizontal bar, some kind of bodyweight suspension kit, or even a rope and door anchor attached at the top of a door.
- Position yourself so that you are holding your chosen piece of exercise kit with your hands just past shoulder width apart.
- Your arms should be fully extended with a slight bend in your elbows.
- Keeping your back flat, abs, core and glutes engaged, walk your feet so that your lower body is forward of your hands.

Movement

- As you exhale, pull your elbows back so that your upper body moves towards your hands.
- Once at the top of the movement, your hands should be in line with your mid chest.
- Keep your abs, core and glutes engaged throughout the movement.
- Do not round your shoulders or back and ensure to maintain the

body alignment that you started with.

- Once at the top of the movement, inhale as you return to the start position.

Extra info

Although this is an early progression for pull ups, it can be challenging for many people. It is an excellent exercise provided that it's done correctly. Being aware that this is an exercise to strengthen the latissimus dorsi, rear deltoids and traps is key. To ensure this, think "shoulders back and down". Study the illustration and make sure you are in the same position at the top of the movement.

You can make this exercise less challenging by reducing the angle that you start from. Likewise, the more parallel to the floor you can perform this exercise, the more challenging it will become.

2nd progression – Engage and hang

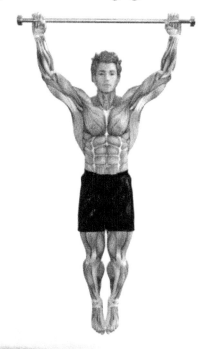

Start position

- You will need a pull-up bar or an equivalent piece of kit.
- Your hands should grip the bar so that they are just past the line of your outer shoulders.
- Engage your core and glutes.
- Engage your traps and lats by pulling your shoulders slightly back and down, whilst also slightly pulling your elbows down. This will create a slight bend in the elbows.
- Keep your head facing forward or looking up slightly.

Movement

- This can be used as an isometric exercise so the start position can be held for as long as possible before a short rest and another set.

- The exercises can also be used as an isotonic exercise. To do this, count reps from the act of trap, lat engagement, and the elbow bend.

Extra info

This exercise is the start of a pull up and will serve to condition the essential muscles that are used for full pull ups. Try to perfect this start position with the isometric method and focus on holding this for at least 10 seconds before moving onto the isotonic version.

3rd progression Standard pullups

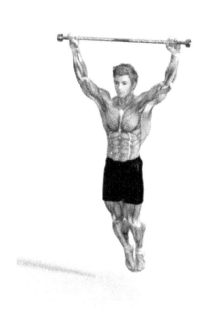
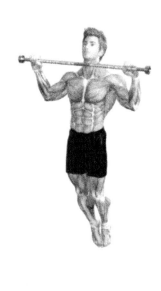

Start position

- You will need a pull-up bar or an equivalent piece of kit.
- Your hands should grip the bar so that they are just past the line of your outer shoulders.
- Engage your core and glutes.
- Engage your traps and lats by pulling your shoulders slightly back and down, whilst also slightly pulling your elbows down. This will create a slight bend in the elbows.
- Keep your head facing forward or looking up slightly.

Movement

- Keep your core and glutes engaged as you pull your elbows down towards your sides. This will bring your upper chest closer to the bar.

- Keep your head looking slightly up or directly forward.
- Ensure that you simultaneously pull your shoulders back and down to engage your traps and lats as you bend your elbows.
- Exhale as you lift your weight and inhale when returning to the starting position.

Extra info

This may seem like a big jump from the previous progression, but it really is the next step aside from assisted pull ups. Assisted pullups are ok but people tend to get stuck on a plateau while using the assisted version. I believe negatives are a much better option if you are struggling to progress from the previous progression to this one. To that end, if you can perform the previous progression competently, consider "negative reps" of this exercise. This is explained earlier in the book in the "negatives & eccentric training" chapter.

Dips Progression

The dip is a compound exercise that puts a big workload on the triceps. Other muscle groups used to perform a dip are the pectorals, anterior deltoids, and rhomboids.

For some instructors, dips are a controversial exercise, and it's apparent why. A well-performed dip from a trainer that has a good foundation of muscular conditioning is likely to be beneficial for that trainers fitness progression.

If, however, a trainer performs dips with slight problems with their exercise form, they can put a significant amount of strain on the shoulder joint, which can lead to long-term injury.

This is something to remember with dips. If you have pain in your shoulders, reassess your exercise form, see a physio or a good personal trainer to look at any mistakes you may be making. Exercise form is important with all movements, but a slight misalignment with dips has the potential to cause big problems.

1ˢᵗ progression - Assisted dips

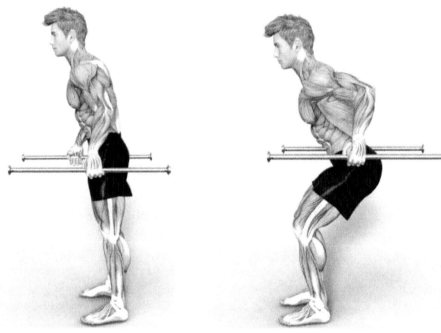

Start position

- You will need a set of dips bars or equivalent pieces of exercise kit. Two sturdy chairs will work.
- Position your dips bars so that when gripped, they are slightly past shoulder width apart.
- Stand between the bars and take a grip so that your hands are forward of your hips.
- Keep your back flat, look forward and hinge slightly at the hips to position yourself as shown in the first illustration.
- Try to take the weight of your body on through your triceps and chest.
- Keep your core engaged and keep your head facing forward.

Movement

- As you inhale, bend your elbows to lower your body. Allow them to flare out slightly, but not too much. Aim to lower yourself so that your upper arms are parallel to the floor.
- Once at the top of movement, exhale as you return to the start position.
- Keep your core engaged and back flat throughout the exercise.

Extra info

As we are using our legs as stabilisers with this exercise, it's important to use them as just that and not rely on them. We want to develop our triceps and chest with this exercise, so the less we use our legs, the quicker we will develop. The range of movement is important in this exercise as it's a personal thing. The bigger the range of movement, the better, but we should also be aware of our own limits. Dips is a controversial exercise as it puts a lot of stress on the shoulders, so it's best to play it on the side of caution and only lower to where you feel comfortable regarding shoulder mobility.

2nd progression -Seated dips

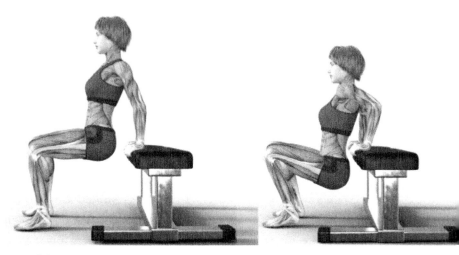

Start position

- You will need a bench or equivalent. A sturdy chair that won't slip is a good option.
- Place your hands on the bench slightly past shoulder width with your fingers facing forward.
- Take your body weight onto your triceps as you assume a seated position.
- Your feet should be at a distance away from the bench so that your upper legs are parallel with the floor.
- Keep your back flat, your core, abs and glutes engaged and your head facing forward.

Movement

- As you inhale, lower your upper body by bending your elbows.
- Allow your elbows to flare out slightly as you lower.
- Once you are at your maximum range of motion, exhale and return to the start position.
- Try to focus the workload onto your triceps and keep your head up,

core and glutes engaged throughout the exercise.

Extra info

If you feel strain on your shoulders in the start position, try widening your hand spacing. Keeping your head in a neutral position will help with your alignment. Be aware of leaning forward or rounding your back in this movement. Remember that we want the workload to be on our triceps.

3rd progression - Standard dips

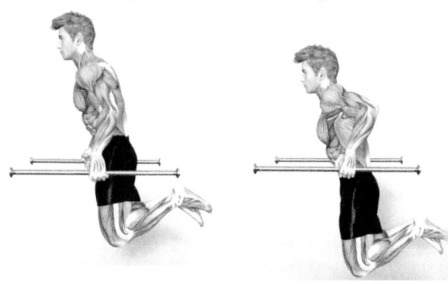

Start position

- You will need a set of dips bars or equivalent pieces of exercise kit. Two sturdy chairs will work.
- Position your dips bars so that when gripped, they are slightly past shoulder width apart.
- Stand between the bars and take a grip so that your hands are forward of your hips.
- Keep your back flat, abs and core engaged, and look forward as you take the weight of your body by lifting your legs.

Movement

- As you inhale, bend your elbows to lower your body. Allow them to flare out slightly, but not too much. Aim to lower yourself so that your upper arms are parallel to the floor.
- Once at the top of movement, exhale as you return to the start position.
- Keep your core engaged and back flat throughout the exercise.

Extra info

When lifting your legs to take your bodyweight, you may find it useful to cross your ankles behind you. This may make your position feel more stable.

If you find your shoulder is strained at the start position, try moving the dips bars wider. It's really important to remember here that range of movement is good but not at the expense of shoulder health, so be cautious.

Shoulder Press Progression

The shoulder press is a compound exercise that targets the deltoids. Other muscles that are used for a shoulder press are the trapezius and triceps.

Exercises for progressive shoulder press advancement have a slight cross over with those of the chest press progression.

Full bodyweight shoulder press is a challenge for many people as the more advanced variations of the exercise require strong, well-conditioned deltoids along with confidence to perform the exercise. The theory behind shoulder press progression relies on an increased incline of press, essentially from a push-up position, and this is where the crossover appears.

If you are working towards push-up progression, you are technically working towards shoulder press progression and vice versa.

1ˢᵗ progression - Standing, incline press

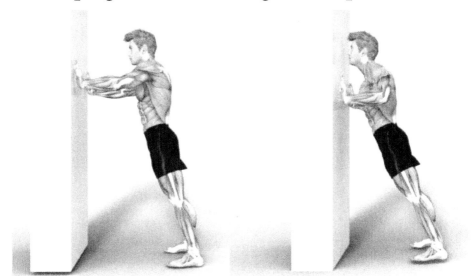

Start position

- Find a solid, upright surface to work with. A straight wall is ideal.
- Position your hands on the wall so your arms are parallel to the floor and in line with your mid chest.
- Make sure your hands are spaced so that your thumbs are in line with your outer shoulder.
- Take a step backwards so that you are taking the weight of your body.
- Keep your back flat, abs engaged and look forward.

Movement

- As you inhale, bend your arms by lowering your body towards the wall until your nose almost touches the surface.
- Your elbows should flare out only slightly.
- Once at the top of the movement, exhale as you return to the start position. This is one rep.

Extra info

Lowering yourself until your nose touches the surface will serve as a good gauge for maximum range of movement and will help you keep your back straight. Remember that the further you step back while setting up your position, the more challenging it will be, but the more of an incline that you create here will put a bigger workload on the shoulders, so this is your aim when using this exercise for shoulder exercise progression.

2nd progression – Incline press

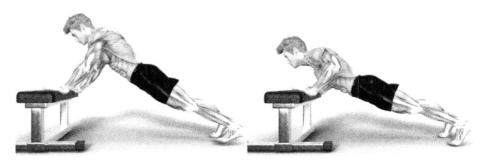

Start position

- You will need a bench or equivalent. A low wall or solid chair can work.
- Position yourself so that your hands are just past shoulder width apart on the bench and inline with your chest.
- Take the weight of your upper body by keeping alignment to form the incline.
- Ensure your back is flat, core and glutes are engaged and your head is in a neutral position facing forward.

Movement

- As you inhale, lower your upper body towards the bench by bending your elbows and allowing them to flare out slightly.
- Ensure that you keep your core engaged and back flat throughout the exercise.
- Once at the top of the movement, as you exhale, push the bench away from you, returning to the start position in a controlled manner.

Extra info

When you reach the top of the movement, ideally, you want the bench to nearly touch your mid-chest. This is a sign that you have a suitable position. If you are struggling to keep your back flat, try looking up slightly as you perform the exercise. It's common to round the shoulders during this movement and this will help to prevent the problem. Another point to note is that the lower the surface that you are working from, the more challenging the exercise will be as this is moving closer to standard push-ups. So if you need a more incremental progression, try using progressively lower platforms.

3rd progression – Pike press

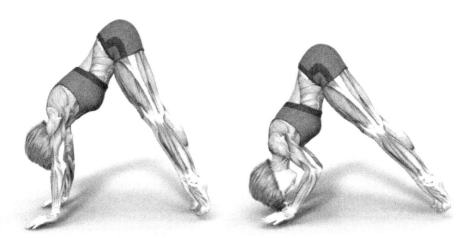

Start position

- Place your hands and feet on the floor by hinging at the hips. Your feet can be flat or you can shift your weight to your toes.
- Walk your hands towards your feet to form a "V" shape with your body.
- Your hands should be just past shoulder width apart and arms straight with a slight bend at the elbows.
- Your legs can be straight with a slight bend at the knees or slightly bent.
- Keep your back flat, abs and core engaged and head in a neutral position.

Movement

- As you inhale, slowly and under control, lower your upper body by bending your elbows.
- Allow your elbows to flare out slightly and stop just as your head is about to make contact with the floor.
- Once at the top of movement, return to the start position as you

exhale.

- Your back should be flat, abs, and glutes should be engaged throughout the movement.

Extra info

The angle of this exercise makes it a shoulder exercise, so the more acute the angle that you can create with the front of your body for this exercise, the more it will benefit your shoulders.

If you struggle with tight hamstrings, this is a good time to simultaneously stretch them out, but be aware of your form if you are going to do this. It is possible to perform this exercise with bent legs, but again, be aware of your posture.

If you find that this is too challenging, simply walk your hands back out slightly, but be aware that the more obtuse the angle you create with the front of your body, the less the workload will be on the shoulders and the more will be transferred to the chest.

4th progression – Elevated pike press

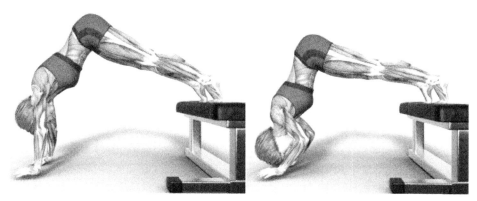

Start position

- You will need a bench, a chair or another type of solid, elevated platform.
- Assume a push up position and place your feet on the bench.
- Your legs should be straight and locked in this position with a slight bend in the knees.
- Keeping your core engaged and back flat, walk your hands towards the bench, hinging at the hips.
- Hand spacing should be just past shoulder width apart, arms should be straight with a slight bend in the elbows.

Movement

- As you inhale, slowly and under control, lower your upper body by bending your elbows.
- Allow your elbows to flare out slightly and stop just as your head is about to make contact with the floor.
- Once at the top of movement, return to the start position as you exhale.
- Your back should be flat, abs, and glutes should be engaged throughout the movement.

Extra info

There are a few incremental things you can do to make this exercise more challenging. If you find it too difficult, don't walk your hands back as far to reach the starting point. This will make the angle smaller, but be aware that this is designed to be an exercise to develop the shoulder muscles, so too small an angle will move the workload onto the chest muscles.

To make this more challenging, you can move your hands closer to the bench or increase the elevation by using a higher bench. If you continue to progress and increase the elevation of your feet, you will find the next progression to be a more seamless transition.

5th progression – Standard shoulder press

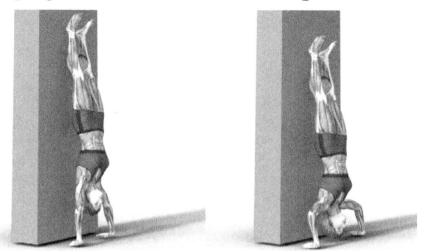

Start position

- You will need a solid, upright surface. A strong wall is perfect.
- Plant your hands on the floor about 12 inches away from the foot of the wall.
- Kick up with your feet to perform a handstand against the wall.
- Once in the handstand position, ensure that your abs, core and glutes are engaged and your body has a straight alignment.
- Keep your legs straight, but slightly bent at the knees. The heels of your feet should rest against the wall.
- Your elbows should not be locked out, but should have a slight bend whilst taking your bodyweight.

Movement

- As you inhale, slowly and under control, lower your upper body by bending your elbows.
- Allow your elbows to flare out slightly and stop just as your head is about to make contact with the floor.
- Once at the top of movement, return to the start position as you

exhale.

- Your back should be flat, abs, and glutes should be engaged, your legs should be straight and the heels of your feet should remain in contact with the wall throughout the movement.

Extra info

This is an advanced exercise but should be very accessible for those who can perform the previous progression competently, especially if using a higher platform elevation.

To get into the start, position requires a certain amount of confidence, however. If you are ready for this exercise but struggling with the start position, consider making your next goal to attain an isometric hold of this movement. Practice the "kick off" with a friend and have them guide your feet towards the wall.

Once you master this exercise, you can even use paralletts or push up bars for extra range of movement.

Bodyweight Squats Progression

The squat is a compound exercise that targets the quadriceps. As the squat is a big compound movement, the exercise also uses the hamstrings, gluteus maximus and the calves when performed.

Leg training is often overlooked with bodyweight routines, but the legs and glutes are large muscle groups that should never be neglected. As the squat uses large muscles to perform, there are more benefits than simple muscular conditioning. It's true that all other resistance exercises raise the heart rate and burn calories when performed, but the squat is especially good at this.

Standard, bodyweight squats are a great exercise for everyone and they can be the limit of progression in most people's exercise routines. Progressions after this, such as pistol squats, are very specialist and are out of reach for some trainers. If you have knee problems, for instance, I would advise that pistol squats are approached with extreme caution or left out altogether.

1st progression - Seat squats

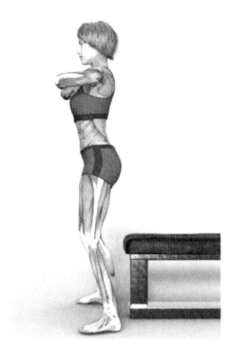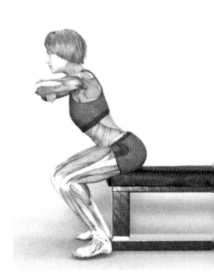

Start position

- You will need a bench or an ordinary household chair.
- Stand with your back flat, abs and core engaged. Your feet should be about shoulder width apart and head in a neutral position.
- Fold your arms across your chest, ensuring your upper arm is parallel to the ground or have your arms straight out in front of you parallel to the ground.
- Ensure that the chair or bench is behind you and underneath your glutes.

Movement

- As you inhale, lower yourself towards the chair, bending at the hips and knees.
- Keep your heels in contact with the floor.

- Keep your back flat, head in the neutral position and upper arms parallel with the floor.
- At the point that your glutes just touch the bench, this is the top of movement. Once here, exhale as you return to the start position.

Extra info

This exercise can be used in everyday life when sitting on any chair. This is a great way for beginners to familiarise themselves with the exercise. When using this in a workout, the idea of the bench or chair is for a depth gauge and, more importantly, to offer reassurance against falling backwards.

To get the most benefit from this exercise, you should never take the workload off by actually sitting down. Concentrate on squatting until you lightly touch the surface with your glutes, then return to the start position.

2nd progression - Bodyweight squats

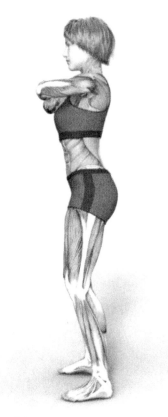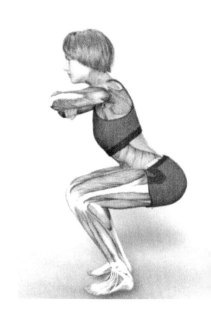

Start position

- Stand with your back flat, abs and core engaged. Your feet should be about shoulder width apart and head in a neutral position.
- Fold your arms across your chest, ensuring your upper arm is parallel to the ground or have your arms straight out in front of you parallel to the ground.

Movement

- As you inhale, lower yourself by bending at the hips and knees.
- Keep your heels in contact with the floor.

- Keep your back flat, head in the neutral position and upper arms parallel with the floor.
- At the point that your quads are parallel with the floor, this is the top of movement. Once here, exhale as you return to the start position.

Extra info

This is exactly the same exercise as the previous progression. The only difference is that there is no bench for reassurance. The progression may seem like a subtle one, but it's significant in that being able to perform bodyweight squats without a bench will give you a bigger range of movement, meaning more muscle engagement and more confidence in further progressions.

3rd progression – Elevated pistol squats

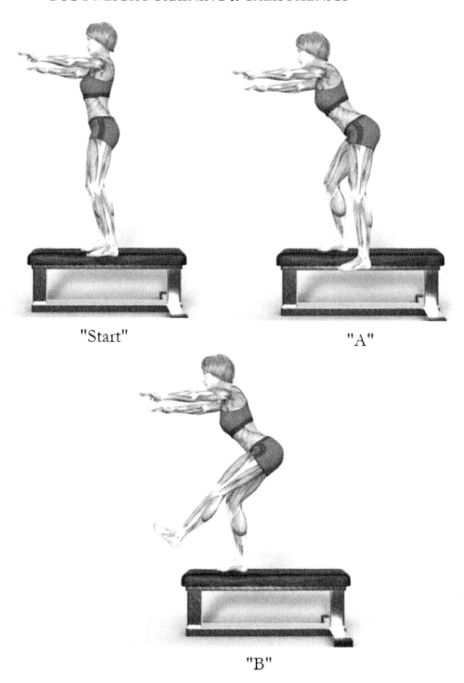

"Start"

"A"

"B"

Start position

- You will need a sturdy bench or elevated platform.
- Balance on the bench with one foot planted and the other hanging over the side. All of your bodyweight will be supported by the leg of the planted foot.
- Have your arms straight out in front of you, parallel to the ground.
- Stand with your back flat, abs and core engaged, and head in a neutral position.

Movement "A"

- As you inhale, lower your body towards the floor by bending at the hip and knee of your working leg.
- Keep your hips aligned, abs and core engaged, arms parallel to the floor and head in the neutral position.
- Squat down until the point that you are about to lose balance or your trailing foot is about to touch the floor.
- Once at the above stage, as you exhale, return to the start position.
- Once you can competently perform movement "A" and reach a top of movement and position that puts your trailing foot close to the ground with each rep, move onto movement "B".
- Perform the same exercise with both legs.

Movement "B"

- As you inhale, slowly and under control, swing your trailing leg in a small arc away from your body to position it in front of you.
- The trailing leg should be straight with a slight bend in the knee when in this position.
- Lower your body towards the floor by bending at the hip and knee of your working leg.
- Keep your hips aligned, abs and core engaged, arms parallel to the floor and head in the neutral position.
- Lower yourself to the point that you are about to lose balance, pause

for a second or two and then, as you exhale, return to the start position.

- Perform the same exercise with both legs.

Extra info

This is an advanced exercise and is not advisable for people with hip or knee injuries or other issues relating to these joints.

A common mistake with this exercise is to lose hip alignment by "reaching for the floor" with the trailing leg, so be aware of this throughout the exercise.

When working on the range of movement, it's also important to take your time with this. You, are essentially performing a one legged squat, so it may take a while to develop the range of movement. To speed this along, once you are at the point that you are about to lose balance, hold this position for several seconds before returning to the start position. This will build up your muscle strength at that point so you can attempt to reach a lower position in future training sessions.

4th progression – Pistol squats

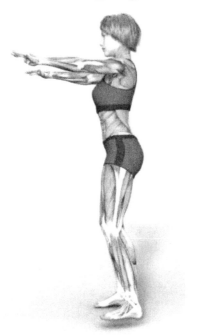
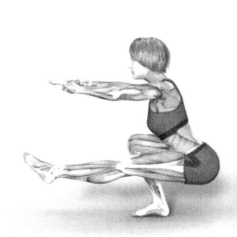

Start position

- Stand with your back flat, abs and core engaged. Your feet should be about shoulder width apart and head in a neutral position.
- Have your arms straight out in front of you and parallel to the ground.
- Stand with your back flat, abs and core engaged, and head in a neutral position.

Movement

- As you inhale, slowly and under control, swing your trailing leg in a small arc away from your body to position it in front of you.
- As you perform the above step, lower your body towards the floor by bending at the hip and knee of your working leg.
- The trailing leg should move to a forward position as you perform the

squat. The lower you progress into the squat, the more forward and parallel with the floor this leg should become.

- Keep your hips aligned, abs and core engaged, arms parallel to the floor and head in the neutral position.
- Lower yourself to the point that you are about to lose balance, pause for a second or two and then, as you exhale, return to the start position.
- Perform the same exercise with both legs.

Extra info

This is highly advanced move that takes a lot of practice and muscular development to achieve. Technique is as important as the muscular development with this one, so prolonged, consistent development of the previous progression may be required.

If you are having trouble keeping balance, try widening the arc of your trailing leg, bringing your arms out towards your sides slightly, or both. If you move your arm position, ensure that they stay parallel with the floor.

As with the previous progressions, ensure that you focus on your hip alignment, but try to reach a deeper squat position in each training session, pausing at your limit to develop muscular stability.

Abdominal & lower back exercises

This is a guide to effective resistance training with a focus on full body workouts. So I have included some abdominal and lower back exercises.

If you are training with a resistance routine, and you are performing the exercises with good form, you will engage your abdominal muscles through every rep of every set for all the exercises choices. This promotes core strength and good posture.

Exercises that directly target the abdominals can be used to further strengthen these muscles. When targeting the abs with specific exercises, they should always be among the last exercises in your training session. This is because they are used as support and stabilisation for all other exercises and you don't want them to be fatigued early in your training session.

The same goes for lower back movements. Lower back muscles can be strengthened and conditioned with specific exercises. Lower back pain is a very common problem and, in most cases, strong lower back muscles and good lower back mobility can prevent this. So consider adding a lower back exercise or two to the end of your routine.

Upper abs

1st progression – Seated crunch

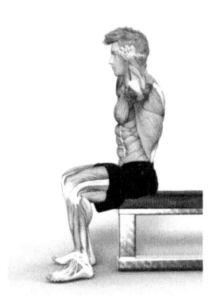 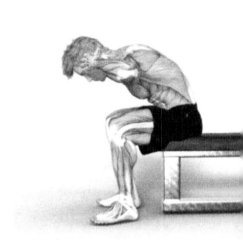

Start position

- You will need a bench or sturdy chair.
- Sit on the bench so that your back is flat, abs are engaged, your head is in the neutral position, your feet are flat on the floor and they are just past shoulder width apart.
- Bring your arms up and place your fingers on your temples.

Movement

- As you exhale, hinge at your hips and round your back to "crunch" your abdominal muscles.
- Keep your feet flat on the floor, head in the neutral position and shoulders remaining back and down.
- Once at the top of the movement, inhale and return to the start position.

Extra info

Breathing correctly in every exercise is important, but with abdominal exercises in particular, the correct breathing pattern will help the movement significantly. Exhaling while performing the crunch will actually start the exercise for you. Remember not to round your shoulders and to keep your feet planted on the floor.

2nd progression – Crunches, wrists to knees

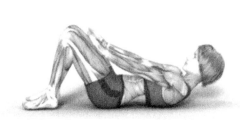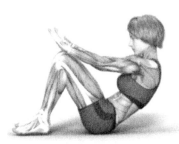

Start position

- Lay flat on the floor so your back, the back of your head and backs of your legs make full contact.
- Bring your knees up towards your chest by putting both feet flat on the floor. Keep your knees together. Your heels should be close to your glutes.
- Lift your head and shoulders off the floor by engaging your abdominals.
- Straighten your arms so that your palms are flat against the front of your quads.
- With your abdominals engaged, tilt your hips slightly to push your lower back into the floor.

Movement

- As you exhale, arch your back to "crunch" your abdominal muscles.
- Keep your arms straight, but slide your palms down your quads until your wrists are in contact with your knees.
- Once at the top of movement, inhale and return to the start, position

under control.

Extra info

One of the more common mistakes with abdominal exercises is not observing the "hip tilt". A good set of crunches will maintain lower back contact with the floor. This will not only protect the lower back, but it will engage deep core muscles and offer a much more efficient abdominal workout.

When returning to the start position between reps, it may be tempting to put your head and shoulders back on the floor, but this should be avoided. If the start position is relaxed, the tension will be lost from the abdominal muscles, causing a dilution of the set.

The "wrist to knees" part of this exercise is predominantly a gauge for range of movement. It's a relatively small movement, but this depth gauge can help beginner trainers with the familiarisation of abdominal engagement and prep for future progressions.

3rd progression – Crunches, fingers on temples

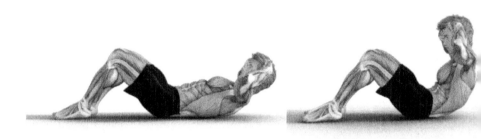

Start position

- Lay flat on the floor so your back, the back of your head and backs of your legs make full contact.
- Bring your knees up towards your chest by putting both feet flat on the floor.
- Lift your head and shoulders off the floor by engaging your abdominals.
- Bring your arms elbows up so that your fingers are resting on your temples.
- With your abdominals engaged, tilt your hips slightly to push your lower back into the floor.

Movement

- As you exhale, arch your back to "crunch" your abdominal muscles.
- Keep your feet firmly planted on the floor and lower back in contact with the floor.
- Keep your head in the neutral position and fingers on your temples.
- Once at the top of movement, inhale and return to the start, position

under control.

Extra info

With this exercise as a progression from the previous, we have no "depth gauge" so you should aim for maximum contraction of your abdominal muscles whilst being conscious of your lower back in contact with the floor. This may take some practice to become comfortable with, but it is an important part of abdominal and core development.

When working towards maximum range of movement, it is common to tuck the chin or bring the elbows towards the midline of the body. This will cause loss of form and alignment and dilute the workload. So be aware of this too.

4th progression – Crunches on exercise ball

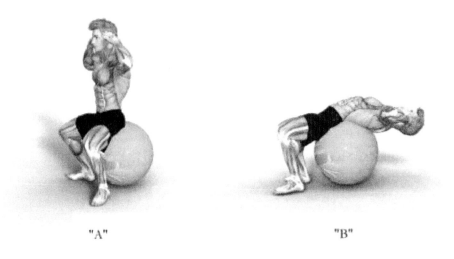

"A"   "B"

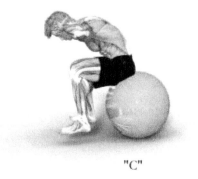

"C"

Start position "A"

- You will need an exercise ball.
- Sit on the exercise ball so that your back is flat, abs are engaged, your head is in the neutral position, your feet are flat on the floor and they are just past shoulder width apart.
- Bring your arms up and place your fingers on your temples.

Movement "B"

- As you inhale, hinge at the hips to lean backwards over the ball.
- Whilst leaning backwards, if needed, walk your feet forward, allowing the ball to roll up your back.
- Once the ball is resting in the small of your back, plant your feet and lean back further to hyperextend your back slightly.
- You should feel the stretch on your abdominals.

Movement "C"

- As you exhale, arch your back to "crunch" your abdominal muscles.
- Keep your feet firmly planted on the floor.
- Keep your head in the neutral position and fingers on your temples.
- Once at the top of movement, inhale and return to the start, position under control.

Extra info

This exercise does require a specific piece of exercise kit, but it is excellent to use as a full range of motion movement.

If you decide to add this to your exercise routine and have trouble balancing on the ball, widening your feet should help with this. If you want to make this more challenging, bring your feet closer together.

5th progression – Crunches feet raised

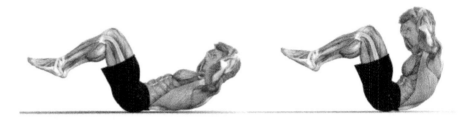

Start position

- Lay flat on the floor and bring your knees up towards your chest, bringing your feet into an elevated position.
- Lift your head and shoulders off the floor by engaging your abdominals.
- Bring your arms elbows up so that your fingers are resting on your temples.
- With your abdominals engaged, tilt your hips slightly to push your lower back into the floor.

Movement

- As you exhale, arch your back to "crunch" your abdominal muscles.
- Keep your feet elevated and lower back in contact with the floor.
- Keep your head in the neutral position and fingers on your temples.
- Once at the top of movement, inhale and return to the start, position under control.

Extra info

This can be a challenging upgrade for many people. If you are finding the progression too tough, try holding the start position and use it as an isometric exercise. Concentrate on the hip tilt that pushes your lower back into the floor whilst making sure that your feet are stable in the elevated position.

Once you get comfortable with this, try smaller crunch movements rather than a full crunch and work towards range of movement progression in future workouts.

6th progression – V Sit

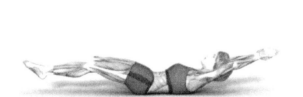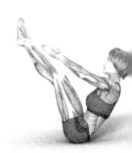

Start position

- Lay flat on the floor keeping your legs straight and together, but ensure to maintain a small bend in the knees.
- Tilt your hips slightly to push your lower back into the floor.
- Engage your abdominals and glutes and lift your heels off the floor about an inch.
- Lift your head and shoulders off the floor while keeping your abdominals engaged.
- Bring your arms up so that they are straight with a slight bend in the elbows above your head.

Movement

- As you exhale, roll your upper body off the floor whilst simultaneously raising your legs.
- Keep your arms straight with a slight bend at the elbows forward, towards your feet.
- Your leg lock position should also be maintained and head in the neutral position.
- Ensure that your abdominals and glutes are engaged throughout the movement.

- Once you have formed a "V" shape with your body and you are balancing on your glutes, this is the top of movement. Inhale and return to the start position under control.

Extra info

This is an advanced movement and should only be attempted by trainers that have a strong core. A common mistake with this exercise is to use momentum to perform the movement; this significantly reduces the intended training effect. The exercise should be performed under control with strict form.

Also, it is important to keep your shoulder alignment with this exercise. It can be tempting to "reach" with your arms towards your feet, causing rounding of the shoulders. The last thing to note with this exercise is that when returning to the start position, you should always maintain.

If you become competent at this exercise and would like a further challenge, when at the top of the movement, try pausing for a second or two before returning to the start position.

Lower abs

1st progression – Lying knee raise, single leg

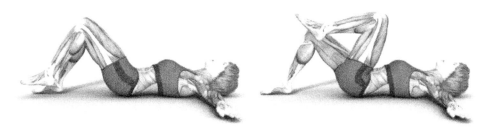

Start position

- Lay flat on the floor, have your legs bent so your feet are flat to the floor and about hip width apart.
- Tilt your hips slightly to push your lower back into the floor.
- Engage your abdominals and glutes and lift one foot about an inch off the floor. This will be the "moving leg."
- Place your arms out to your sides, palms down and flat to the floor for stability.
- Ensure that your head and back are in contact with the floor throughout the movement.

Movement

- As you exhale, raise your "moving leg" up towards your chest until your lower leg is parallel with the floor.
- Your knees should remain at the same angel as the starting position.
- The position of your head, back and arms should be maintained throughout the movement.
- Once you are at the top of the movement, inhale and return to the start position.
- When you have completed the planned reps for this exercise, repeat for the other leg.

Extra info

When returning to the start position with this exercise, you should not return the foot of the "moving leg" back to the floor, always maintain a small gap.

Be conscious of lower back position and keep awareness of hip alignment. Once fatigue starts to kick in, it may be tempting for one side of your lower back or glutes to lift off the floor. If you feel this happening, fix it immediately, or finish the exercise if it is indeed due to fatigue.

2nd progression – Double knee raise

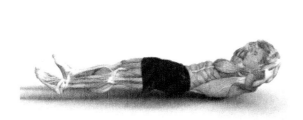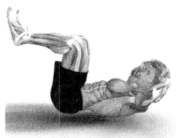

Start position

- Lay flat on the floor, keeping your legs straight and feet about hip width apart.
- Tilt your hips slightly to push your lower back into the floor.
- Engage your abdominals and glutes and lift both feet about an inch off the floor.
- Bring your head and shoulders off the floor to engage your abdominals.
- Raise your arms and hands to place your fingers on your temples.

Movement

- As you exhale, raise both legs up towards your chest whilst also bending your knees, until your lower legs are parallel with the floor.
- The position of your head, back and arms should be maintained throughout the movement.
- Once you are at the top of the movement, inhale and return to the start position.

Extra info

If you find this is too much of a progression, you can change the tart position slightly by keeping your head and back flat to the floor and placing your arms out to your sides, palms down and flat to the floor for stability. This is the same upper body starting position as the previous progression.

It's also important for this exercise to be aware of using momentum to perform the movement. It can be tempting to "bounce" or "jolt" your legs to kick-start the movement. We want to avoid this, as it can dilute the workload from our target muscle groups.

3rd progression – Leg raise

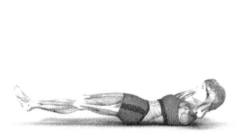 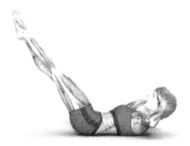

Start position

- Lay flat on the floor, keeping your legs straight and close together.
- Tilt your hips slightly to push your lower back into the floor.
- Engage your abdominals and glutes and lift both feet about an inch off the floor.
- Bring your head and shoulders off the floor to engage your abdominals.
- Raise your arms and hands to place your fingers on your temples.

Movement

- As you exhale, raise both legs up towards your chest, keeping them straight. You should stop just before your legs are vertical.
- The position of your head, back and arms should be maintained throughout the movement.
- Once you are at the top of the movement, inhale and return to the start position.

Extra info

With this progression, there will be a bigger temptation to use momentum to perform the movement than the previous one, so, again, be aware. Also, you can also place your arms and head on the floor for stability if you find this to be too much of a progression from the previous exercise. If you choose this option, be aware that it will be much easier to lose your lower back stability by pulling it away from the floor.

4th progression Seated knee raise

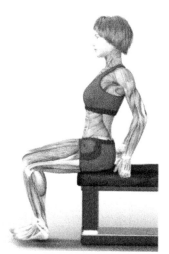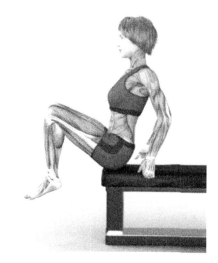

Start position

- You will need a bench, strong chair or equivalent.
- Sit on the bench so that your back is flat, abs are engaged, your head is in the neutral position.
- Your legs and feet should be together and lifted off the floor slightly.
- Grip the sides of the bench with your palms facing in.

Movement

- As you exhale, lift your knees towards your chest.
- Ensure that you maintain a flat back and natural head position.
- Once your upper legs reach a 45-degree angle, this is the top of the movement.
- Inhale and return to the starting position.

Extra info

Again, be aware of using momentum, but with this exercise, there may be temptation to arch your back and bring your shoulders forward to complete the movement. Always keep your back flat, abs and glutes engaged and use your grip on the bench for stability if this happens.

Remember when returning to the start position to keep your feet about an inch away from the floor. This will keep tension in the abdominals and give a more efficient workout.

5th progression Hanging Knee raise

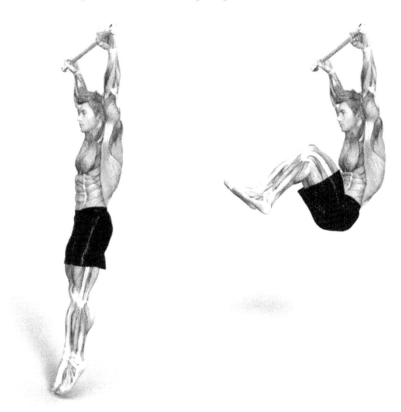

Start position

- You will need a pull-up bar or an equivalent piece of kit.
- Your hands should grip the bar so that they are just past the line of your outer shoulders.
- Have your feet and knees together, legs straight, but maintain a slight bend in the knees.
- Engage your core and glutes to bring your legs forward slightly.
- Engage your traps and lats by pulling your shoulders slightly back and down, whilst also slightly pulling your elbows down. This will create a slight bend in the elbows.
- Keep your head facing forward or looking up slightly.

Movement

- As you exhale, bend your knees slightly to tuck your lower legs. Bring your legs up towards your chest until your quads form a 45-degree angle with your upper body.
- Ensure that you hinge at the hips to fully engage the lower abdominals.
- Once at the top of movement, inhale and return to the start, position under control.

Extra info

As you tuck your lower legs, it may be tempting to use the momentum to complete the movement. To avoid this, you may want to tuck your legs before you start the movement. But tucking your lower legs as you perform the movement will help towards the next progression. The longer that your legs stay straight, the more that this exercise looks like the next progression. This is an exercise that helps to practise as technique plays a part, so have a practice, but remember the fundamentals and what the exercise is designed to do.

6th progression Hanging leg raise

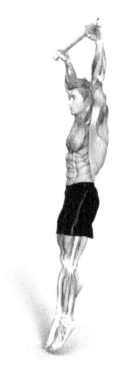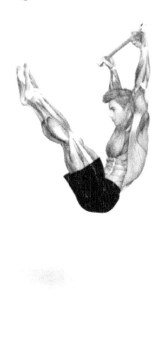

Start position

- You will need a pull-up bar or an equivalent piece of kit.
- Your hands should grip the bar so that they are just past the line of your outer shoulders.
- Have your feet and knees together, legs straight, but maintain a slight bend in the knees.
- Engage your core and glutes to bring your legs forward slightly.
- Engage your traps and lats by pulling your shoulders slightly back and down, whilst also slightly pulling your elbows down. This will create a slight bend in the elbows.
- Keep your head facing forward or looking up slightly.

Movement

- As you exhale, bring your legs up towards your chest until they form a 45-degree angle with your upper body.
- Maintain the start position for your lower legs and upper body.
- Ensure that you hinge at the hips to fully engage the lower abdominals.
- Once at the top of movement, inhale and return to the start, position under control.

Extra info

If you find that this is too much of a progression, you can complete the exercise with bent legs. If you choose to do this, bend your legs at the knee to tuck your lower legs at the start of the movement. Maintain this leg position throughout the movement.

To ensure that you get the most value from this exercise, concentrate on control, both on the leg elevation and when returning to the start position.

When reaching the top of movement, ensure that you are aiming for maximum contraction. Your hips should tilt forward and your lower back should be rounded. This is the benchmark.

Lower back

The stabiliser

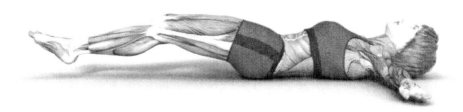

Start position

- Lay flat on the floor, keeping your legs straight, feet together and flat on the floor.
- Tilt your hips slightly to push your lower back into the floor.
- Engage your abdominals and glutes and lift one foot about an inch off the floor. This will be the "moving leg".
- Place your arms out to your sides, palms down and flat to the floor for stability.
- Ensure that your head and back are in contact with the floor throughout the movement.

Movement

- This is an isometric hold and should be used based on the individual's ability.
- Ensure to maintain glute and abdominal engagement throughout the hold.
- Breathing should be slow and controlled throughout the hold.

Extra info

This exercise engages the lower abs and lower back. To make this effective for lower back stability, focus on keeping your glutes engaged and your lower back pushed into the floor by tilting your hips.

Double leg bridge

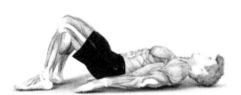 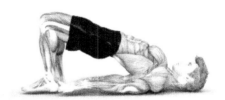

Start position

- Lay flat on your back, bring your knees up towards your chest by putting both feet flat on the floor about shoulder width apart.
- Ensure that your head back and arms are in contact with the floor.
- Your arms should be by your sides or out to your sides slightly for stability.

Movement

- As you exhale, engage your glutes and push through your heels to bring your lower body away from the floor.
- Once you have raised your body up to form a straight line from your knees to your chin, this is the top of the movement.
- Once you reach the top of the movement, as you inhale, return to the start position under control.

Extra info

This is a great exercise for the lower back and glutes. The major points to note on this are to always push through your heels and to note the top of movement position. It's unnecessary to bridge further than the point that the front of your body forms a straight line from your chin to your knees. After this point, your back will be in "hyper extension".

Hyper extension is not always a bad thing, but on this exercise, there is no need to incorporate the movement.

Alternate swim

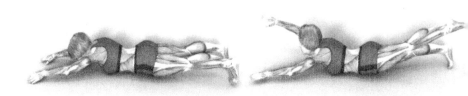

Start position

- Lay flat on your front with your arms outstretched above your head.
- Your head should be in the neutral position. If this is uncomfortable, lift your head slightly so your chin is in contact with the floor.
- Place the tops of your feet flat to the floor or plant your feet with your toes.

Movement

- Engage your abdominals and glutes.
- As you exhale, lift your left arm away from the floor as you lift your right leg away from the floor.
- Inhale and return to the start position.
- Pause for a second or two.
- As you exhale, lift your right arm away from the floor as you lift your left leg away from the floor.

Extra info

It's important to remember that the movements used in this exercise are small ones and that they need to be performed under strict control.

There should always be a slight pause between alternations and the start position re-established. This will help to prevent any miss-alignment issues that could occur if the movement was continuous.

Dorsal raise

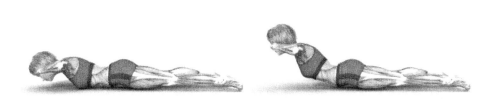

Start position

- Lay flat on the floor with your head in the neutral position.
- The tops of your feet should be in contact with the floor and your legs straight.
- Bring your arms up and to your sides, placing your fingers on your temples.
- Engage your core and glutes and lift your head slightly away from the floor.

Movement

- As you exhale, lift your upper body away from the floor.
- Keep your glutes engaged.
- Keep your feet in contact with the floor.
- Keep your arms in the start position.
- Only raise your upper body to where you feel the tension.
- Once at the top of movement, inhale and return to the start position.

Extra info

This is another small movement, and there is an element of back hyper extension. So it's really important to keep this movement slow, controlled and smooth. If this is a new exercise, approach it with caution and test your range of movement abilities.

There is no need to over extend on this, you can benefit from small movements and the engagement alone.

Superhero

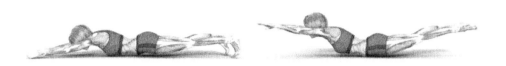

Start position

- Lay flat on your front with your arms outstretched above your head.
- Your arms and legs should be slightly bent, but locked in this position.
- Place the tops of your feet flat to the floor.
- Your head should be in the neutral position. If this is uncomfortable, lift your head slightly so your chin is in contact with the floor.
- Engage your glutes and core as you lift your arms and legs slightly away from the floor.

Movement

- As you exhale, lift your upper body and lower body away from the floor.
- Keep your glutes engaged.
- Only raise your body to where you feel the tension.
- Once at the top of movement, inhale as you return to the start position.

Extra info

This is another lower back exercise that requires extra caution. Make sure that you only extend to where you are comfortable with. Always keep your glutes engaged and always make sure you perform this with slow and controlled movements.

Single leg bridge

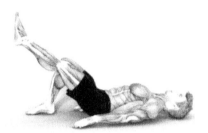 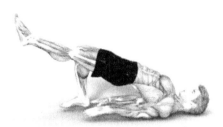

Start position

- Lay on your back, keeping your legs straight and feet about hip width apart and flat to the floor.
- Tilt your hips slightly to push your lower back into the floor.
- Engage your abdominals and glutes, lift and straighten one leg. Ensure you lock the leg but keep a slight bend in the knee.
- Place your arms out to your sides, palms down and flat to the floor for stability.
- Ensure that your head and back are in contact with the floor throughout the movement.

Movement

- As you exhale, engage your glutes and push through your heel to bring your lower body away from the floor.
- Your raised leg should remain fixed in place throughout the movement.
- Once you have raised your body up to form a straight line from your knees to your chin, this is the top of the movement.
- Once you reach the top of the movement, as you inhale, return to the start position under control.
- When you have completed the planned amount of reps with one leg

raised, raise the other leg and repeat the process.

Extra info

As we are only using one leg planted on the floor, this will significantly encourage the possibility of miss alignment in our lower back. It is really important therefore to ensure that our glutes are fully engaged and stable before we start each repetition.

This exercise is an advanced move, as it's only advisable to perform once there is a good amount of condition and strength in the lower back muscles from previous exercise progressions to counteract the imbalance of the raised leg.

It's also very important to keep this exercise movement slow, smooth and controlled.

Cat cow

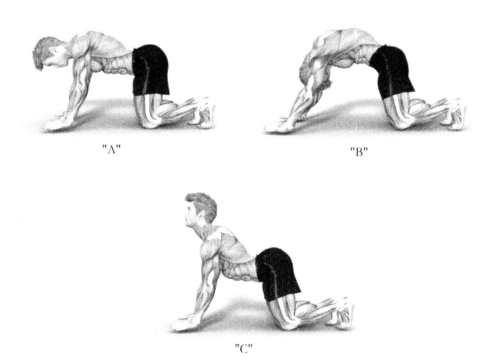

"A"

"B"

"C"

Start position "A"

- Position yourself on all fours so that your knees and palms are contacting the floor.
- You should have a slight bend in your elbows, your head should be in the neutral position and your knees are directly beneath your hips.
- Your palms should be beneath your shoulders and toes, contacting the floor.

Movement "B"

- As you exhale, drop your head towards your chest, arch your back and tilt your hips forward.

- Keep your palms, toes and knees fixed in position.
- Whilst performing this movement, keep your abs and glutes engaged.
- Once you reach the top of movement, as you inhale, return to the start position ("A").

Movement "C"

- As you exhale, tilt your hips backwards whilst moving your head to look upwards.
- Keep your palms, toes and knees fixed in position.
- Once you reach the top of movement, as you inhale, return to the start position ("A").

Extra info

This exercise is used for mobility and a stretch for the lower back and is often prescribed to people who are recovering from lower back pain or injury. Although this is the case, it is an excellent movement to incorporate into your routine that's relevant for all levels of fitness.

It is important to note that this exercise should be performed in a slow, smooth, and controlled manner.

Thank you! If you found this useful, I'd like to help further...

First off, I would like to thank you for your purchase. It really means a lot that you spent your time on this guide. I am a self-published author with a passion for training and helping people get to where they want to be with fitness and by reading; you are supporting me and fuelling my passion.

This guide should give you a brilliant start in the world of bodyweight training and the planning that goes with it. But this is not my first fitness book! I've been writing and self-publishing for several years. I've written books on fitness motivation, planning, bodybuilding, home workouts and long distance running. These guides are based on my experience and formal education.

I've been a long distance endurance runner, a competing bodybuilder, and I have worked with personal training clients to change their lives through fitness, so I have a lot to share.

If you found this short guide useful and would like to read more about body transformations, fitness motivation, home workouts or more about resistance training and would like a clear path to follow, I have plenty more for you to look at including workbooks and journals for you to plan and track!

Most of my books are available in eBook and paperback format, and some are also available as audio titles narrated by an exceptional voice actor called Matt Addis.

Each fitness book is written as a standalone guide but also has its place as part of a series. So if you are a total beginner and want to become a bodybuilder or marathon runner as an end goal, I have you covered! Jump in at the start of the series with *"Fitness & Exercise Motivation"* and follow the steps, I'll be at the starting blocks with you and we will cross the finish line together!

If you would like to learn more about this series and my other books, you can do so by visiting my author page. Visit Amazon and search "James Atkinson", you will see my ugly mug, click it, and you should be taken to my page. Alternatively, just follow the link below - ☺

James Atkinson Author Page[1]

---

1. https://www.amazon.com/James-Atkinson/e/B00EN9HZ48/ref=dp_byline_cont_pop_ebooks_1

As we all know, diet plays a big part in health and fitness, and the two subjects fit hand in hand. So I would like to offer you a free download of seven healthy recipes that I created and use regularly myself. You can copy the recipes exactly, add your own twist to them, or simply take inspiration from them.

If you would like to grab this, you can do so by following the link below.

jimshealthandmuscle.com/
healthy-recipes-sign-up/[2]

Remember The Podcast!

Trying to create an online business is tough, especially in the fitness niche! There is a lot of noise, "fairy-tale" fitness supplements, big personalities, and celebrities with huge online followings pushing their fitness ideas that often drown out the information that will actually make the difference.

In an attempt to widen my online reach, I created a podcast that is designed for the beginner who really wants to get results from their efforts. I set out to create bite sized podcast episodes of around twenty minutes that gave honest, actionable advice to the listener. This is still in its early stages, but I have to say that I've absolutely loved doing these podcast episodes and it is something that I plan to get stuck into more in the future.

If you are interested in fitness podcasts, you can find mine at

AudioFitTest.com[1]

Or search Audiofittest wherever you get your podcasts from.

It would be great to have you along! If you do stop by, I would also really appreciate "Likes", "follows" and reviews. These things really help! The same goes for Amazon reviews for the books. If you have chance and you found the book useful, it would mean the world to me if you left a star rating and a short review.

Thanks again for your support and I wish you all the best with your training. Remember, I am always happy to help where I can, so if you have any questions, just give me a shout!

All the best,

Jim

I will leave you with a bit about cardio training ☺ ...

Cardio Training.

This is an excerpt from one of my other books – *"Marathon training & Distance Running Tips"*. It's a book that's designed to take the beginner from their first thought of running right up to the finish of a marathon. Running is not just about putting your trainers on and getting out there to cover mileage, there is a lot more involved, from mind-set, to running posture, from motivation to preventing blisters. So if you are looking to start running, or even want to start cardio for weight loss, this will almost certainly help.

Here is an excerpt from the book. I hope you enjoy it and find it useful.

CHAPTER 7 - *Marathon Training & Distance Running Tips*

WHERE TO START

This section is really aimed at the beginner, but it may still hold some useful information for the veteran.

With anything that you do, you have to start from the beginning, and I firmly believe that having a solid foundation to build on is a must if you want results.

It would be great if every goal that you had was achievable overnight, but with any serious fitness goal, the mind-set of progression training is a fundamental factor for success!

Of course, you would not expect to be able to run a marathon in a few short weeks of training. And I would like to clarify that if you are just starting out, there is a long road ahead of you... (Excuse the pun.)

This may sound negative, and many people would be put off by the fact that at least six months of hard, consistent, and smart training will only get them a small step closer to their goal.

I'm talking about the guys that have never done any exercise before and would like to take up the challenge of a marathon.

If you are this guy or gal, I would first like to congratulate you on making this decision and also like to reassure you that you CAN do this.

When you cross that finish line, I'm sure that it will be one of the greatest accomplishments of your life, and your training, character building, and determination leading up to this accomplishment will definitely enrich you as a person.

YOUR FIRST RUN (WHAT TO EXPECT)

The first time you step out of your door, you will probably be motivated, have some shiny new running shoes and training attire, and be ready to start pounding the pavement.

There are a few things that can literally kill your motivation and make you hang up your new running shoes permanently if you are not careful. The biggest killer of your goals in this situation is...

"too much, too soon."

I have seen it, overheard conversations about it, and actually been there myself.

Everything's great. You are all ready to start your marathon training. You have planned your route, you are hydrated, and you know this is going to be the start of something very special! You give a few cursory hamstring stretches and set off on your first run.

Two minutes in and you are fighting for air, your lungs are on fire, you feel sick, and you are wondering how on god's green earth you are even going to finish your first run when you are in this state and you can still see your front door?

Believe me; if you have never felt this way before, you need to actually be there to understand the mental effect that this has on you. It can be devastating!

You will no doubt be able to relate to this feeling very soon as your training progresses. But I will say that it can be controlled, and when you look back at these events, they won't seem that bad. It's just while you are there that you will feel your world is ending!

Before you start your training, please read the Breathing and Running Style chapters. If you can understand and practice this before you even start your first run, it will help you out massively.

YOUR FIRST RUN (WHAT TO DO)

Once you have your breathing and running style sorted, you will be ready for your first run.

The thing is, your first run will not actually be a run! Remember that this is all about progression and you have to start somewhere. If you have never been on a run before, your body isn't used to the kind of stresses put on it, so you will probably end up in the state that we just talked about.

Once you have your route planned out, you should don your trainers and get ready, as you would expect. But your first training session should be a steady walk around your route. This will benefit you more than you probably think.

First of all, it will start you on your routine. Next, it will get you used to your new running shoes. These are a vital piece of kit for any runner.

"Bad shoes = Bad feet, and with bad feet, you can't do a whole lot of running"

Another thing that walking your route will help you with is getting your body used to prolonged activity. These early sessions will also help you to prepare mentally for your training too as you will be able to visualise your route and you will get to know how long this will take you or how close you are to the finish line.

Depending on how fit you are or how quickly you progress, you may want to do this walk for the first full week, but you can assess your progress after your first session.

All that being said, starting off slowly is one thing, but progression is vital if you want to improve and actually reach "long-distance runner status."

This "easy start" approach may be refreshing to some readers, but you also need to progress and push yourself. It may take you a few weeks to find your limits and assess your fitness progression, but this is all part of the process. It is important that you find the right balance.

This is what I would do if I had never done any fitness:

First Session

• Walk my route at a consistent pace

Second Session

• If the previous session was too easy, I would pick up my pace a bit.

• If the previous session was too hard, I would shorten the route a bit.

• If the previous session made me out of breath slightly and had me sweating but I was otherwise comfortable, I would consider a short jogging stint at the last section of my next session.

As you can see, there are a few factors that you can change each time that you train. The important part at this stage is to never sit back and go through the motions; you MUST be progressing. If your sessions do not push you slightly, you will not develop the endurance that you are looking for.

But at this point, there is no need to get to the stage of physical discomfort mentioned at the beginning of this chapter. It will only mess with your mind.

Also by James Atkinson

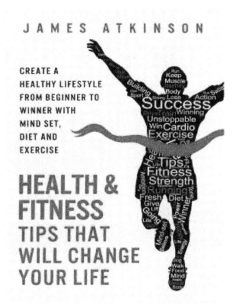

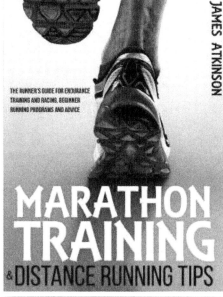

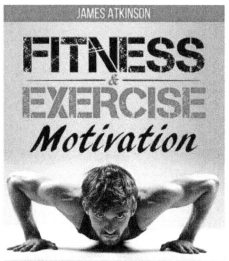

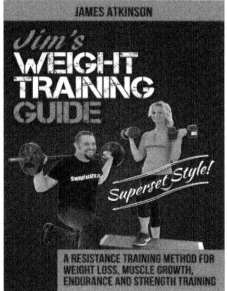

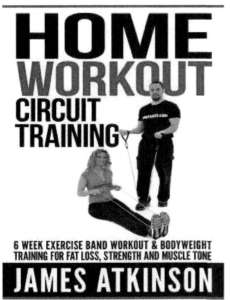

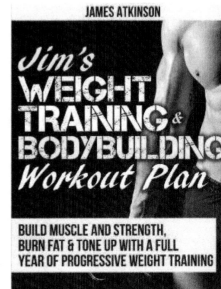

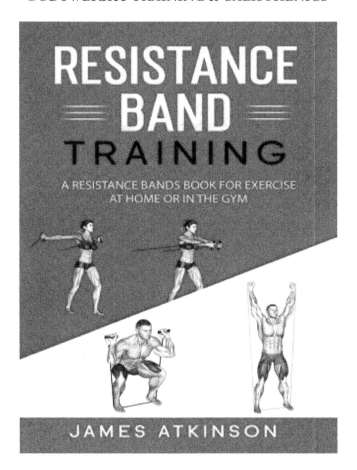

Blank Program Cards

BODYWEIGHT TRAINING			

ROUTINE #		

EXERCISE	SETS	REPS	TIME

WEEKS	MON	TUE	WED	THURS	FRI	SAT	SUN
1							
2							
3							
4							
5							

BODYWEIGHT TRAINING			

ROUTINE #			

EXERCISE	SETS	REPS	TIME

WEEKS	MON	TUE	WED	THURS	FRI	SAT	SUN
1							
2							
3							
4							
5							

BODYWEIGHT TRAINING			

ROUTINE #			

EXERCISE	SETS	REPS	TIME

WEEKS	MON	TUE	WED	THURS	FRI	SAT	SUN
1							
2							
3							
4							
5							

BODYWEIGHT TRAINING			

ROUTINE #		

EXERCISE	SETS	REPS	TIME

WEEKS	MON	TUE	WED	THURS	FRI	SAT	SUN
1							
2							
3							
4							
5							

BODYWEIGHT TRAINING			
ROUTINE #			

EXERCISE	SETS	REPS	TIME

WEEKS	MON	TUE	WED	THURS	FRI	SAT	SUN
1							
2							
3							
4							
5							

BODYWEIGHT TRAINING			

ROUTINE #		

EXERCISE	SETS	REPS	TIME

WEEKS	MON	TUE	WED	THURS	FRI	SAT	SUN
1							
2							
3							
4							
5							

BODYWEIGHT TRAINING			

ROUTINE #	

EXERCISE	SETS	REPS	TIME

WEEKS	MON	TUE	WED	THURS	FRI	SAT	SUN
1							
2							
3							
4							
5							

BODYWEIGHT TRAINING			

ROUTINE #			

EXERCISE	SETS	REPS	TIME

WEEKS	MON	TUE	WED	THURS	FRI	SAT	SUN
1							
2							
3							
4							
5							

Printed in Great Britain
by Amazon

17560570R00106